Doug Depew has written the most complete "how to and what for" book on orthodontic treatment. A must-read for anyone on the path to happy, healthier and more beautiful smiles.

Myron Guymon, DDS, MS

Logan, UT

Doug Depew is an exemplar for orthodontists all over the world. Change Your Smile, Change Your Life *is a must-read for anyone interested in pursuing orthodontic treatment. This book embodies Doug's humble brilliance and commitment to bettering the orthodontic profession.*

Neal D Kravitz, DMD, MS

South Riding, VA

Dr. Doug Depew cares from his heart for his patients and his staff. His customized orthodontic treatment results in beautiful, healthy smiles for every patient. Dr. Depew invests his staff in continuing education to ensure high-quality care for each patient. Always a leader in the orthodontic profession, Dr. Depew inspires other orthodontists through his Trapezio training school, his speaking and his consulting. Readers of Change Your Smile, Change Your Life *will benefit from Dr. Depew's wisdom about smiles and life!*

Jackie Dorst, RDH, BS

Safe Practices—Instrument Sterilization, Infection Control

and OSHA Safety Consultancy

As an orthodontic clinician and educator for almost fifty years, a former professor of orthodontics, and chairman and graduate program director at four major universities, I've had the privilege of training over 250 of the best and brightest dentists in the country in the specialty of orthodontics. The guiding principle taught to the residents was to provide every patient requiring services with the best available treatment to the highest standard of care. Today, the public is bombarded by marketing techniques that portray people as consumers rather than patients with unique health care needs. In this book, Dr. Depew examines the issues, dispels the myths, and provides clear and practical answers for those considering orthodontic care.

Richard F. Ceen, DDS
Adjunct Professor, Department of Orthodontics,
Texas A&M University, College of Dentistry

Dr. Depew, although only few years older than me, has always been an inspiration for me to work harder and continue to improve myself professionally and in all aspects of life. He's always in search of the newest technology and is a pioneer in implementing the latest in the science of orthodontics in his practice. His office and his team members are like no other, everyone is genuinely pleased to see you and welcome you into their office, which is only a testament of Dr. Depew's character and leadership. In the last twenty-one years of my practice we collaborated on numerous complicated cases and the results were impressive every time. This book is another testament of his dedication to orthodontics and to providing the best treatment to his patients.

Wade A. Diab, DDS, MS
Diplomate of the American Board of Periodontology
Kennesaw, GA

I have had the pleasure of working with many of the best and brightest in orthodontics, and I have not met a more innovative, intelligent, and integrity-focused doctor than Doug Depew. His book is a terrific reference for anyone wanting to learn more about our profession.

Jamie Reynolds, DDS, MS
Rochester Hills, MI

Before I worked with Dr. Depew, I previously worked in other orthodontic offices while I was starting my own practice. They were all different—some cut corners and reflected that in their low price. Others had outstanding results and charged more for their treatment. Dr. Depew's office stood out to me. His office had a desire for attention to detail, quality, honesty, technology and teamwork. To put it simply—he and his staff cared about the quality of care their patients received, and the results showed. This attitude and thought process could be felt by the patient and could be seen through their quality smile.

Mark Causey, DMD
Gainsville, GA

Dr. Depew's expertise, candor, and willingness to listen and understand his patients' concerns is simply exceptional. He is one among the very few in North America whose orthodontic skills make the impossible possible. My atypical and challenging case could only be handled by an exceptional orthodontist like him. His extraordinary professional wit and understanding beats the conventional wisdom that has brought smiles back to people they most deserve . . . and I am one of those lucky ones . . . bravo Dr. Depew!

Ameen Farooq, PhD
Professor of Architecture at KSU

Change Your
Smile,
Change Your
Life

Change Your Smile, Change Your Life

YOUR GUIDE TO Orthodontic Treatment

D. DOUGLAS DEPEW, DMD, MS

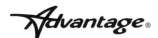

Many of the images herein are from the Dolphin Aquarium patient-education program. For more information, go to www.dolphinimaging.com.

Published by Advantage, Charleston, South Carolina.
Member of Advantage Media Group.

ADVANTAGE is a registered trademark, and the Advantage colophon is a trademark of Advantage Media Group, Inc.

Printed in the United States of America.

10 9 8 7 6 5 4 3 2 1

ISBN: 978-1-59932-999-4
LCCN: 2018962858

Book design by Carly Blake.

Advantage Media Group is proud to be a part of the Tree Neutral® program. Tree Neutral offsets the number of trees consumed in the production and printing of this book by taking proactive steps such as planting trees in direct proportion to the number of trees used to print books. To learn more about Tree Neutral, please visit **www.treeneutral.com**.

Advantage Media Group is a publisher of business, self-improvement, and professional development books and online learning. We help entrepreneurs, business leaders, and professionals share their Stories, Passion, and Knowledge to help others Learn & Grow. Do you have a manuscript or book idea that you would like us to consider for publishing? Please visit **advantagefamily.com** or call **1.866.775.1696**.

To my father, Donald Albert Depew, who taught me the value of hard work. And to my wife, Vicki Depew, for putting up with me and supporting me all these years.

Table of Contents

Foreword

"Who could be calling this late?" my sleepy wife asked. A quick peek at the caller ID revealed a Georgia number, and upon seeing the 770 area code, I recognized it as Doug Depew calling. "Are you going to answer it?" she asked on the second ring, outwardly hoping I'd get it before it rang a third time.

"Ya, I'll get in the other room." We were on Mountain time, whereas Doug was on the east coast—I knew it had to be important if he was calling that late. I picked up the cordless phone and left the room so my wife could get back to sleep. Those were the days of young practices, small children and impossible schedules to keep.

I answered the phone and Doug greeted me with a long drawn out, "Duuude…" I think every conversation we've had has started with the same "Duuude," a favorite greeting between close friends he has perfected with a little southern drawl and just the right amount of that something to remind you he's from Canada as well.

He started, "You've got to look at my website."

No going back to sleep now, I thought, at least not for a while. I paused for a second and took a breath. He assured me he knew what time it was and answered my query that he'd only been on the computer for four to five hours. Pretty much sums up Doug in both passion for the profession and his endless energy expended in a nearly thirty-year career of doing everything he starts better the more he does it.

I first met Doug in New Orleans. We were both interviewing for orthodontic residencies and most of the applicants were in one room waiting for the activities to follow. I think, unconsciously, we were sizing each other up. While most of us were happy to get the interview and were just hoping to get in somewhere, there was this one guy that asked all the right questions and seemed to have all the right answers. Little did I realize what an affect that guy would have on my professional and personal life. We were classmates in the Baylor Orthodontic program for two years and that spawned a lifelong friendship and professional respect that is ongoing.

For years, I kept on my desk a picture of him standing in front of a model trimmer in a lab apron. We worked our way through school by doing lab work. The picture was one I took at about two o'clock in the morning on a Wednesday after we'd been there most of the only evening we had that week to tackle the work. All that work was due Thursday morning—just a few hours later. It was a continual reminder how lucky we are to be orthodontic specialists and what it took to get there. It's certainly been worth it now, looking back when fatigue was so constant we just accepted it as normal.

In the early years of our career, continuing education was a little harder to come by than in the digital world we live in now. We would meet at AAO annual sessions and attend lectures at the Southern and Georgia orthodontic association meetings. We'd scout the exhibit halls looking for that one next thing that would make our lives and practices so much better. We'd share a room and split the costs. Budgets were tight, but we both felt the importance of keeping up and learning more. That led to opportunities to talk for hours on what the new "stuff" was and how we were going to incorporate it when we got back home to our practices. Doug was, is and will always be about quality patient care. Early on, he mastered the tooth moving mechanics and then set a course to improve the quality of the patient experience in his offices. While many would have just coasted with their mastery, Doug has continued to learn and master the new technologies in both patient care and practice management. More importantly, he's shared what he's learned.

Many years ago, Doug recognized the need for an orderly and consistent orthodontic assistant training system. Not finding any that suited him, he made it his life work to develop a program that has made him the world leader in auxiliary training. Unsurprising to me, he did the same thing to the undergraduate orthodontic clinical materials while we were still in residency. We've long ago quit trying to meet up and spend time together at the AAO meetings—he's way too involved with lectures, staff workshops or telling people about his AAO endorsed Trapezio training programs.

More than that, he's a good man and great friend. He and Vicki have raised a wonderful family. We both got lucky when our wives became the same kind of friends we'd become and supported each other those long days of residency when it was common to spend eighteen to twenty hours together and away from them. We've planned and executed nearly every year a "trip of a lifetime." African Safaris, fishing in Guatemala, trips into the Rocky Mountains on my horses, it never gets old.

Lest you think it's all fun and games, on one trip we forbid Doug to bring his laptop computer. He wasn't to work on anything orthodontic that trip. It was supposed to be a vacation. He just brought a book so he could do some light reading and completely devoured a newly printed orthodontic text book on temporary anchorage devices on the long flight. So much for the inflight movies. He had to read a novel for the first time since high school. He was out of orthodontic material for once. I think he outlined a textbook he eventually wrote on the flight home while us lesser men slept.

It just seems legit that he's written a "how to and what for" book on orthodontic treatment. Pay special attention to the directions he gives on finding a qualified orthodontic specialist with your best interests in mind. You can tell he loves what he does and loves what it can do for the amazing people we treat. He's worked a lifetime to improve the whole orthodontic treatment process for both the providers and the recipients. You'll hear words like amazing, visionary, organized, entertaining, and informative spoken about him.

I'm just lucky I guess I get to call him friend and colleague. He just calls me "Duuude." Someday I hope to call him in the middle of the night, wake him up and plant a few seeds of thought that will keep him up all night too. Until then.

Duuude...
Myron Guymon, DDS, MS

Preface

Thank you for picking up *Change Your Smile, Change Your Life: Your Guide to Orthodontic Treatment.* With today's environment of competing priorities—both of our time and financial resources—we all strive to balance needs and wants, and in the end, do what is best for our children and ourselves.

I sincerely feel blessed to work within the field of dentistry and particularly in the specialty of orthodontics. As an orthodontist, my goal is to change lives by helping patients achieve amazing smiles, and enjoy the experience getting there. We have seen personalities blossom, career paths become enriched, and relationships flourish after helping our patients transform their smiles.

I have spent almost a year writing *Change Your Smile, Change Your Life*. It's been tough with so many other things to do in life. The process has made me reflect on why I do what I do. It has made me think introspectively and place myself in the shoes of the reader, which has helped me understand what you, the reader, would want to know.

In this time where information is readily available at our finger tips, we can find loads of competing information about orthodontics, and often downright misinformation. Finding the best orthodontist and the right care for yourself or your child can be confusing. My goal in this book is to set the record straight.

In *Change Your Smile, Change Your Life*, I explain the benefits of orthodontic treatment, some of the more common philosophies and methods used, and how to find the orthodontist that is right for you and your family. I also discuss all of the new technologies that have made treatment faster, more comfortable, and more affordable. I also discuss important things to know about during treatment and the importance of retainers once you have finished.

I hope you find the pages in this book helpful. Although you may wish to read the entire book, it is set-up as a reference so you can read the parts that are most pertinent to you. There are plenty of images that may help you in understanding some of the unique terminology found in orthodontics.

Happy reading!

Acknowledgments

This written work in *Change Your Smile, Change Your Life* was a long time coming. There is so much that went in to its making. There is no way I could have done it myself. So many people have influenced me in arriving at the contents of this book—many unknowingly. While some had a direct impact on the book, many had more of an indirect influence. Some were instrumental during the writing process, while others helped get me to the point where I could undertake this project.

I would first like to acknowledge the doctors and staff at both Baylor College of Dentistry and the Medical College of Georgia School of Dentistry for believing in me and helping me reach a point where I could work in this incredible profession. In particular, professors Dr. Richard Ceen, Dr. Peter Buschang, and Dr. Rohit Sachdeva put all their efforts into teaching me and my fellow residents all they could to help us better serve our patients. My favorite clinical instructor was Dr. Monte Collins, who took a day each week out of his own private practice to come share his knowledge with us. He was a great example to us all. My co-residents were also great friends and examples, including Dr. Myron Guymon who wrote the foreword for this book.

As this book is intended as a guide to orthodontic treatment, I had to think back to all the many conversations I've had with patients and parents about their questions, concerns, comments, and compliments. It helped me understand what was important to them and what they appreciated. You know, over the years, I have had so many thoughts, phrases, and explanations I have used in discussing orthodontic treatment with patients, parents, and those I am teaching and privileged to be in front of giving lectures. This book puts many of those conversations into written form. So even though there is not one specific person, I will say thank you to all these folks for making me think on my feet.

My team at the office played a role by giving me ideas for some of the content, by reviewing some of the drafts of the book, and offering alternatives. Particular thanks goes to Dr. Kristen Hall and Kenneth Moss. But most of all, I appreciate the team for just putting up with me as my mind was often on the book rather than what they felt I should be doing. The team also was instrumental in narrowing down the cover design as we had many options from which to choose.

I am particularly grateful to my loving wife, Vicki. Without her support and encouragement this book would not have been possible, nor would the family atmosphere we've established at Depew Orthodontics. She aids me in staying grounded and focused. She was particularly helpful in her assistance in finalizing the book cover design and some of the ideas within the book. I must also include my three children Andrew, Ashley, and Ryan for bringing me and Mom such great joy and making us proud. I love you all.

I'd like to acknowledge Conner, Katie, and Tiffany for posing for the photo on the cover and Chrissi Higham for her photographic expertise.

Orthodontics—It's About the Experience

As an orthodontist, I love to see people smile. I love seeing the change that comes over people as their treatment helps them have a beautiful, healthy smile. For many people, orthodontics can really be a life-changing experience.

But orthodontics is about far more than creating smiles. It's about the overall experience—the environment in which you are treated and the friendships you make along the way. Orthodontic treatment involves a long-term doctor-patient relationship, so it's important to make the right choice in providers.

With so many different technologies today, and so many providers to choose from, it's important to find someone who will give you the level of care you deserve. Because when it comes to orthodontics, a lot of confusion is being created by inaccurate, conflicting, and often deceptive information from multiple sources: Facebook, the Internet, advertisements, well-meaning friends, nonprofessional and professional blogs, and YouTube videos. People are also confused by the fact that treatments and techniques vary among orthodontists. And there's even more confusion about having treatment done by a general dentist versus an orthodontist.

My goal is to help clear the air and give you accurate information about orthodontics, some of the latest treatments available, and what you should look for when choosing a provider for you and your family.

Orthodontics is complex, but as an orthodontic specialist with nearly three decades of experience, someone who has successfully completed well over fifteen thousand cases, I want to help you understand how orthodontics can change your life and how to get the most out of your orthodontic journey.

Being an orthodontist is the best job in the world. I get to work with wonderful people—team members and patients who genuinely want to make each other happy and improve each other's lives. And we have fun—lots of it. On an average day, I see dozens of patients in my practice. I spend my days working with a great team and, together, we help people feel better about themselves and help them achieve fantastic smiles and healthy bites. When I'm not seeing patients, I'm digitally designing new smiles, evaluating teeth, measuring facial structure, and projecting tooth movement. My team and I also spend a lot of time talking with parents about their child who is receiving treatment, and with potential patients about the options available to them. We want to share our knowledge and to inform people so that they feel comfortable about their treatment, and about treatment options. It's a very upbeat, fun environment with music playing, a lot of high-fiving, and lots of humor. In short, it's hard not to smile when you visit our practice.

Make no mistake. We work hard. That's something I learned from my father, Donald Depew, who taught me that reward comes from a job well done. We moved quite a bit when I was young—all over the United States and Canada, but primarily, up and down the east coast. In one of those locations, we lived on a small farm where Saturdays were not play days; they were work days. Besides chores, there was always a project of some sort to be done—building a barn, finishing basements, bailing hay, and more—and it felt great to finish them, one after another, as if I had really accomplished something. I also spent the summers of my younger teen years working on a dairy farm, and in my later teen years, on a ranch in Alberta. I liked to be busy, both physically and mentally. I liked the challenge of figuring out how to finish something I had started. We moved to Georgia when I was a teen, but every summer I returned to Canada to work on my uncle's ranch. Today, when I'm not working in someone's mouth as an orthodontist, I still love being outdoors, camping, skiing, hiking, fishing, golf, or driving a tractor around my farm where I raise and train quarter horses.

Being very active as a youth, I had a few accidents that damaged several of my teeth. By the time I was eighteen, I had undergone treatment to repair eleven teeth, including my front teeth.

But I have good memories of those trips to the dentist and orthodontist. My orthodontist was the father of one of my schoolmates, a man who was very active in the community and whose work ethic and lifestyle I admired when I was growing up. He loved his work, but he understood that family and fun were important, and that his work enabled him to spend time on those other priorities.

By the time I started college, I knew I wanted to work in health care, but, at that time, instead of considering orthodontics, I planned to be a veterinarian. I was in the program long enough to discover that being a veterinarian meant working long days and being on-call, so I decided to look into other areas of health care. That's when I turned to orthodontics. I really wanted a rewarding career in which I could help patients, be involved with kids, and yet set my own hours and be my own boss. It was important to me to be an entrepreneur, to build a business and watch it grow. So orthodontics was a great fit.

After earning a bachelor's degree in microbiology from the University of Georgia, I went to dental school at the Medical College of Georgia. Dental school is tough: thirty-five credit hours at a time, studying for what seems to be twenty-four hours a day. It's college on steroids.

Still, I was number one in my class all of my four years in dental school. That gave me a good shot at being accepted into orthodontic school, which is very competitive: only one or two of the top graduates from dental school are accepted. I applied to seven orthodontic programs and was accepted into three, finally choosing to attend Baylor College of Dentistry in Dallas, Texas. There, I trained for two years, earning a certificate in orthodontics from Baylor College of Dentistry and a master's degree in oral biology from Baylor University. Working closely with my four coresidents and some great instructors, I learned the secrets of creating awesome smiles.

In addition to my school load, I was busy getting married and having kids. To support my family while I was in school, a classmate and I spent our nights making retainers for a couple of local orthodontists. That night work gave me an edge. As I worked on those models, I really studied the teeth and got a lot of practice making retainers. Today, I'm still pretty critical of the retainers and other appliances that come back from the labs I use. It's not uncommon for me to send back an appliance for rework until it fits the needs of my patient.

I remember one patient in particular during my dental school years. Mabel was a woman in her seventies who needed a complete set of dentures. When she first came in, she was, frankly, a pretty grumpy person. But after receiving her new false teeth, she not only had a beautiful smile but also went out and got a complete makeover: new hairstyle, new clothes, and makeup. She even got a new boyfriend! Getting a new smile was the first step in completely transforming her life. From that point on, I knew that my work would be impactful.

Now, orthodontics is very different from the rest of dentistry: the terminology, equipment, supplies, and so on, are completely different. So even with dental training, orthodontic school can be very confusing at first because there is so much to absorb quickly. But a professor told a group of us that even though it was overwhelming, one day "it will all click." He was right, but that happened shortly after graduation. I had joined another orthodontist in his practice, with the intention of taking it over at some future point, but not long after I came onboard, he decided to retire.

Those first couple of years on my own were pretty tough. The practice was busy, but it had been in a bit of a maintenance mode for some time. The patient relationships and the level of care were not what I had envisioned for my own practice. I spent those first couple of years turning that established practice into my own.

The practice had two offices that were not great locations. So, in the office, as sort of a game, I hung a map of the county and had patients place a pin to show where they lived. After a couple of months, I added pins to the map representing the schools and the locations of other dental and orthodontic practices. Once all those pins were placed, I could very clearly see where I needed to relocate the practice: Kennesaw. In the end, only six families actually had to travel farther to get to the newly built office. The office is located in the historic district and is actually on the site of Camp McDonald, a Civil War Confederate training base.

After that move, the practice really grew. I had reached out to schools and businesses, trying to let everyone know that we wanted to be involved in the community. I joined numerous boards and committees and spent a lot of time involved in the local business association, scouting, and soccer club. Several years later, we built a second office serving both Acworth and Dallas, Georgia. It was an especially attractive building on a main road and it still garners a lot of attention. As I write this book, the two practices employ seventeen people, and an associate doctor also sees patients. We're a leading provider of Incognito braces, SmartClip appliances, and Invisalign clear aligners.

Being on the cutting edge with technology is one reason for Depew Orthodontics' success. I'm an early adopter for numerous companies, which gives me access to some of the latest advances. In this ever-changing industry, I want the best for my patients—and of course, for the practice. Although newer and bigger isn't always better, if a technology offers greater efficiency and comfort, then it's something we consider bringing in for those we are privileged to call our patients.

Highly trained and friendly staff have also helped make the practice a success. That's due in part to Trapezio, a training program I developed in the late 1990s as a way of ensuring that assistants on our fast-growing team were trained to industry standards. Back then, there was no real training available for orthodontic assistants, and on-the-job training was time-consuming, inconsistent, and ineffective. The program originally consisted of a course taught in our office, on nonpatient days, to people who wanted to work as an orthodontic assistant and were either local or traveled from other parts of the United States and Canada. Today, the course is primarily web based, the main clients being doctors using it as a training system for their staff. We have also added courses for most positions in orthodontic practice, making our program a training system for the entire practice. Periodic hands-on courses for clinical assistants are offered in our home office or remotely.

The program's comprehensive, standardized training has made me a sought-after speaker and educator of orthodontists and their teams on topics including clinical efficiency, techniques, insurance coding, technological advances, and practice management.

Depew Orthodontics is also the go-to provider for area dentists and their families. Why? Because, like all our patients, they recognize there is something extra to a Depew Smile. That something extra is the artistry behind the smile—and that comes with experience. When patients' braces come off, I am excited because I know that the smile we created will be with them when they receive good grades in school, when they land their first job, when they get married, when they kiss their children—all those great moments in life.

Since orthodontics is part of the medical field, it's viewed as a science. It involves understanding the anatomy of the teeth and gums and how the body functions at the cellular level. We have to understand the growth and development of the body's systems, and how the work we do can affect the whole body. So yes, science is an important part of orthodontics.

But all the science in the world doesn't ensure a great smile without an artistic eye guiding treatment. That's what results in a Depew Smile. Patients wearing a Depew Smile have a signature piece of art. The art of that smile is in the details, something I'll share with you in the pages ahead.

Again, orthodontics is far more than just fixing crooked teeth. Read on and you'll see the difference that training and experience makes; it can literally change your life.

CHAPTER ONE

Transforming Smiles, Enriching Lives

One of the best experiences in the world is seeing the life of a patient transformed through orthodontic treatment. It's exciting to turn a mouthful of less-than-ideal teeth into a healthy, radiant smile for a lifetime. That's what happened to Maria.

When Maria came in for an evaluation, she was just entering her teen years. At that time, she had typical *snaggleteeth*—canine, or eye teeth, that are higher than the rest of the upper teeth and look like a set of "fangs." The rest of Maria's teeth were crooked from overcrowding, and her upper and lower jaws didn't match when she bit down because her upper jaw was too narrow.

The condition of her teeth got her teased a lot at school, so much so that she had taken to covering her mouth when she laughed or smiled. She had become so self-conscious that it had begun to affect her personality. She became an introvert when she was around anyone but her family and closest friends.

At her first appointment, she seemed to be very sad—until we told her that we could help her get a beautiful smile. Then she really lit up. She couldn't wait to get treatment started.

We started by widening her upper jaw with an expansion appliance, which took about two months. Then we put her in SmartClip metal braces with bands that aligned her upper and lower jaws to help her bite fit together properly. She was a great patient, doing her part to ensure that her treatment was a success—she kept her teeth clean, wore her bands and changed them twice a day, and kept all of her appointments.

Over the next two years, we watched Maria transform into a beautiful girl with a great smile—and even with greater self-confidence and self-esteem.

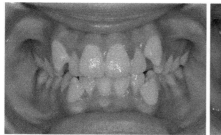
BEFORE

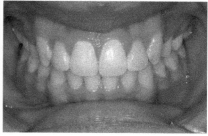
AFTER

FIRST IMPRESSIONS COUNT

Orthodontics is the science of moving teeth into their proper positions and changing the shape of the jaws so the upper and lower rows of teeth fit together properly. But there is so much more to orthodontics than just moving teeth. Much of what doctors and staff do also affects the facial profile, the shape of the face, the fullness of the lips, the ability to speak and swallow properly, even the ability to breathe effectively.

Besides restoring teeth to normal health and function, orthodontics can change perception, leading to a better first impression and better success overall. In fact, a 2012 digital study[1] in which respondents were shown images that had them unknowingly comparing straight teeth with crooked teeth found the following:

- Nearly one-third (29 percent) noticed a person's teeth first.

- Nearly one-quarter (24 percent) said teeth were the one facial feature they remembered most after meeting someone.

- Nearly half (45 percent) perceived a person with straight teeth to be more apt to get a job when going up against someone else with the same skills but with crooked teeth.

- More than half (58 percent) believed people with straight teeth were wealthier and more successful.

- When it comes to dating, more than one-third of respondents said they would not go on a second date with a person who had crooked teeth, and more than half (57 percent) believed that a person with straight teeth would be able to get a date just from their picture.

- Almost three-quarters (73 percent) said a person with a nice smile was more trustworthy.

- More than one-third (38 percent) thought a person with a nice smile was smart.

- Nearly half (47 percent) thought a person with straight teeth was healthier.

Interestingly, the study also found that a majority of the

---

1   "First Impressions Are Everything: New Study Confirms People with Straight Teeth Are Perceived as More Successful, Smarter and Having More Dates," Invisalign, press release, April 19, 2012, PR Newswire, accessed February 16, 2018, https://www.prnewswire.com/news-releases/first-impressions-are-everything-new-study-confirms-people-with-straight-teeth-are-perceived-as-more-successful-smarter-and-having-more-dates-148073735.html.

respondents would give up something for a year if it meant having a nice smile for a lifetime.

Everyone wants a great smile, and an orthodontist is a specialist in making your smile the best it can be. Straight teeth not only look good but also make you healthier. They make you feel great and change how people see you—and how you see yourself.

PATIENT COOPERATION—
THE KEY TO GOOD OUTCOMES

One of my professors had a great saying: orthodontics is the specialty of dentistry in which a *professional* (the doctor) depends on a *juvenile* (young patient) to achieve an *ideal* result. What he meant is that orthodontics is a team effort, and it takes cooperation by everyone on the team to achieve the best result. The orthodontic team alone can't determine outcomes. The patient really is in charge of how well treatment comes out. It's a little like a football team. As the orthodontist, I'm the coach. My assistants are teammates. Parents are cheerleaders who encourage their child to keep going. And the child (or adult patient) is the quarterback, who really is in control on how things turn out.

It's up to the patient to follow the treatment plan to get the desired results. That means:

- Good oral hygiene must be maintained. It is particularly important in orthodontics to brush regularly and effectively because plaque accumulates much faster on teeth that have braces.

- Braces must be kept intact. Hard, sticky, or crunchy foods can break braces. Broken brackets, bands, or wires are not only time consuming to repair and frustrating for the patient—and for the orthodontic team—but also slow down the progress of treatment.

- Auxiliaries must be worn as instructed. If the treatment requires changing out rubber bands, for instance, then it's up to the patient to be diligent if the treatment is going to succeed.

KEEPING TEETH CLEAN

- It is possible and important to floss even when you have braces.
- Brush at least twice a day for at least two minutes.
- Always brush just before going to bed.
- Use a small (pea-sized) amount of toothpaste on your toothbrush.
- Hold the toothbrush at angle to brush above and below the braces wire so bristles go under the wire.
- Use small, circular motions.
- Don't forget to brush along the gum line.
- Additional tools such as oral irrigators, electric brushes, and small interproximal brushes are also really helpful.

Since compliance is so critical to success, in today's busy world we are always on the lookout for ways to make treatment easier on the patient. We consider which treatment will best fit the lifestyle of each individual patient—and yet get the desired results.

For instance, for a young patient who has poor oral hygiene, is reluctant to wear elastics, and whose mom states that he's not so great at following instruction or remembering basic tasks, we consider an option known as a noncompliance appliance: one that is attached 24/7 and does not require elastics.

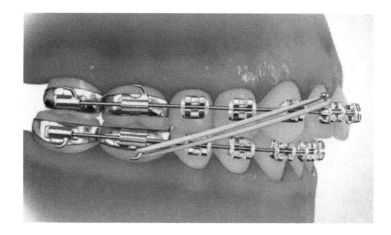

Sometimes patients who we feel will be compliant end up not being so, or they just burn out with treatment. For them, we use attached appliances, as "Plan B." That is what we did with Joel, a twelve-year-old who had crooked teeth and a misaligned bite, as Maria had. We wanted to push Joel's upper teeth backward and his lower teeth forward to decrease his overjet and improve his facial profile. His oral hygiene was borderline when he came in for treatment, but we started him with braces that required him to change out the rubber bands or elastics twice a day. As someone who played sports, he had the discipline to follow instructions. Unfortunately, that didn't transfer to his orthodontic treatment. On a follow-up visit, we found that while his oral hygiene had improved—he was managing to keep the braces clean—he hadn't managed to change his elastics regularly and his treatment wasn't progressing as it should. With his parent's approval, we changed the bands to an appliance that performed the same function but was attached to the braces and required no extra maintenance. That got his treatment back on track.

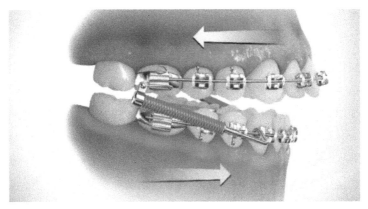

Forsus appliance by 3M

THE SCIENCE OF MOVING TEETH

Moving teeth is both science and art. It is a science because the doctor has to understand biology, histology, physics, geometry, material sciences, engineering, and how those apply to moving teeth. It's an art because it requires the individual judgment, talents, and skills of the doctors (and staff): the experience and eye to customize treatment to create a beautiful, finished smile, a Depew Smile, based on the patient's needs and desires.

The job of the orthodontist and team is to work with Mother Nature—and sometimes against her—to place the teeth and jaws into a better position, functionally and cosmetically. In a growing patient, nature can either help us or hurt us in our efforts. For example, in a patient with an overjet (commonly called overbite), we can harness that growth and focus our efforts on that area to accentuate the growth of the lower jaw to decrease the overjet. However, in a growing patient with an underbite, we have to pull out all the techniques and tools to slow down or even stop that forward growth while the rest of the body catches up with the protrusive lower jaw.

Moving teeth is a process that takes time: gradual movement is essential for lasting change. The natural position of the teeth and bones are influenced by several factors including genetics, muscle pressure, and habits. These can factor into the outcomes of treatment. Let me share with you some of the science basics of what it means to move teeth.

In the mouth, teeth are set in the bone of the jaw. The teeth rest in a "sling"—or what's known as the periodontal ligament—within the socket of the bone. That ligament is made up of small fibers that stretch between the root of the tooth to the wall of the boney socket.

While most people think of bone as something very hard, it is actually a dynamic, ever-changing material. Yes, the enamel of a tooth is permanent—once that outer white shield of enamel is formed, it's there forever. But the bone of the socket, where the teeth live, is always changing, it's always "turning over." That process of turning over is known as remodeling; as old bone breaks down, new bone forms. The remodeling process is what orthodontists use to their advantage to move teeth.

However, the health of a patient's gums also factors into treatment. The gum tissue around teeth and bone must be healthy and stable enough to withstand the movements being made. If the gums are too thin or weak, they can be damaged even more by moving the teeth. And if there is untreated periodontal disease, evidenced by red, swollen gums and loss of bone, as seen on x-rays, initiating orthodontic therapy can make it worse.

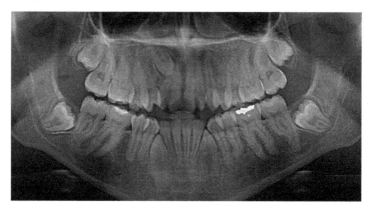

As orthodontic appliances apply pressure to the crown of the tooth—or the part of the tooth that shows outside the gums—the sling space changes. It becomes compressed on the side the tooth is moving toward, leading to loss of bone in that area. The movement causes cells known as osteoclasts to dissolve the bone in that direction of movement. As the bone dissolves, the tooth begins to move into the new space.

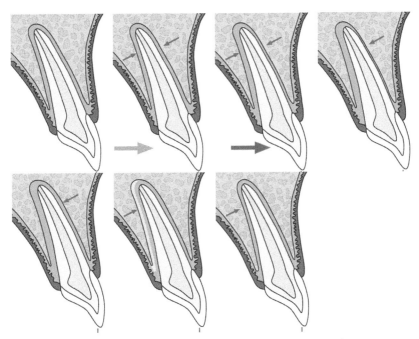

As the tooth moves, bone on one side is compressed,
then resorbs away, and new bone forms on the other side.

Movement also stretches the ligament on the side the tooth is moving away from. That movement stimulates cells known as osteoblasts to create new bone in the socket where the tooth was. However, if pressure applied by the braces was taken away while that new bone was still young, the tooth could easily return to its former position.

There's also a limit to how much teeth can be moved safely. Teeth can only be moved a certain amount in different directions, and the orthodontist and team must understand what those limits are for each patient. Without understanding the parameters for each patient, teeth may quit moving, or even worse, may be pushed beyond the limits of the gum and boney tissue into unhealthy or compromised positions.

Pain tolerance is also factored into treatment. Even though today's braces cause little or no pain, we have to consider just how much discomfort patients can tolerate when figuring out the rate at which to move their teeth.

Bone density can also play a role in how teeth move. The denser the bone, the slower the movement. Bone density varies from person to person, and even varies in different parts of the mouth in the same person. And there are factors that can alter bone density. For instance, teeth move very fast in women who are in their third trimester of pregnancy, while tooth movement is halted by medications such as bisphosphonates, which stop bone from breaking down and are used by people dealing with osteoporosis, a brittle-bone disease.

Like the leader of an orchestra managing many different sections of instruments to ensure a beautiful work of harmonious music, an orthodontist must manage many components in the mouth all at once to ensure a harmonious outcome.

The truth is that, in the right hands, straightening is a much easier process using today's appliances. But treatments are like fingerprints: they are unique to each individual, especially since most patients have more than one problem to address. That's where the artistry comes in.

THE ART OF MOVING TEETH

The planning and finishing of treatment is what separates one orthodontist from another. Planning lays the groundwork for the treatment to come, just as constructing a home or other structure starts with detailed architectural plans. And just as no two artists' works are exactly alike, neither are the finished works of any two orthodontists.

With a Depew Smile, there is a difference, and balance is a key part of it. After thorough planning, creating the perfect balance in a smile begins with positioning the braces and using appropriate technology. Then each smile is looked at as a three-dimensional work of art.

Straight teeth not only look good but also fit together well. When the upper and lower teeth fit together the way they should, it's easier to chew, speak, and swallow. In the ideal finish, the central incisors (middle teeth) on the top are slightly lower than the lateral incisors next to them, for both a pleasing smile and proper function while chewing. The lower edge of the upper teeth follow the curve of the lower lip to form a pleasing crescent. In the ideal finish, the teeth line up in relation to each other, and each tooth is shaped or contoured to look more youthful with edges that have a slight pleasing curve, instead of being totally flat. The upper front teeth are tipped slightly forward in a way that the light reflects upward—for that bit of dazzle. (Front teeth tipped inward don't reflect light well. They tend to look darker and age the face more.) From a front view, however, upper back teeth stand upright outside of the lower back teeth, and the whole smile is wider to fill the mouth so that little or no black corridor shows between the molars and cheek on either side.

Finally, the gum tissue should be healthy and contoured properly to create the perfect balance. Uneven gum tissue or too much tissue over the teeth can be modified so that the gums enhance each tooth's position in the mouth.

As a final touch, we recommend whitening with gel supplied by our office or by the patient's dentist, or with over-the-counter strips.

Here are some of the issues we commonly see and some brief explanations of how we address them from the perspectives of form (appearance) and function:

Crowding refers to overlapping of teeth, where there's just

not enough room for all the teeth. Crowded teeth affect both form and function. When teeth are crowded, they don't look good, but more importantly, they are hard to clean, which can lead to plaque buildup, gum inflammation, periodontal (gum) disease, cavities, and even tooth loss. Treatment involves creating enough room for all the teeth and then lining them up. Crowding is what most people think orthodontic treatment addresses.

Gaps. Although gaps or spaces make it easier to clean your teeth, they can be unsightly. The most common gap occurs between the two front teeth. Gaps are more about form than function. Closing a gap is a matter of positioning the teeth properly.

Missing teeth. There are a number of reasons a person may be missing one or more teeth. Sometimes teeth have been removed because of a fracture or decay. Sometimes it's because of poor oral health that resulted in disease of the gums. Some people have congenitally missing teeth, meaning that they're born without specific teeth—most commonly the upper lateral incisors (second tooth from the center on each side) or the lower second premolars (fifth tooth from center on each side). Missing teeth impact appearance and the person's ability to chew and function well. Treatment for missing teeth involves aligning remaining teeth and either closing remaining spaces or ensuring there is enough space for implants.

Impacted teeth are unable to fully grow into the mouth on their own. Wisdom teeth—the teeth farthest back in the mouth—are the teeth most commonly associated with impaction. But we often see impacted upper canine teeth as well (third tooth from the center). Canine teeth are very important, especially the upper canines, since they are cornerstones and are built and positioned to take heavy chewing forces more than the other front teeth. Often, the timing of their eruption into the mouth occurs when there is not enough room, so they get deflected and develop in a different direction. Treatment involves creating space for them and potentially working with an oral surgeon to uncover them. A small gold chain bonded to the tooth is then used to slowly move that tooth into position.

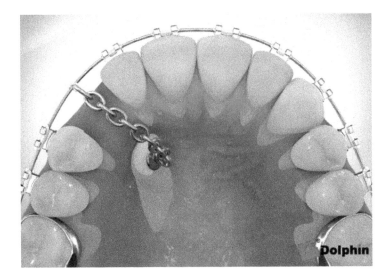

Malocclusion literally means "bad bite." It is a general term used to describe a misaligned bite due to such things as an overbite (top teeth overlapping the bottom teeth excessively), underbite (bottom teeth overlapping the top teeth), and crossbites (teeth tilted inward). Correcting a bad bite can help the patient eat better and be healthier, and it can even alleviate pain symptoms associated with temporomandibular joint (TMJ) dysfunction. Basic malocclusions are discussed further in chapter five.

Excessive or uneven gum tissue makes teeth appear to be longer or shorter than they are. This condition can affect one tooth or several teeth and can often be treated with laser or periodontal treatment to improve appearance and improve gum health.

There is so much more to orthodontics than just straightening teeth, and a successful outcome relies in part on the qualifications of the doctor behind the tools being used.

Compare it to a pilot flying a jetliner: A lot of preplanning and preparation takes place before the plane leaves the gate. The pilot has a long preflight checklist to review. During taxi, takeoff, and ascent, the pilot is at the front of the plane, guiding it into the sky. Once the plane reaches cruising altitude, the pilot can turn over the controls to the copilot or autopilot, and then step back and monitor the flight. As the plane approaches its destination, the pilot then takes over the helm again, ensuring everything is in order to land safely.

Similarly, in orthodontics, the orthodontist does a lot of preplanning and preparation before treatment begins. Once the braces are applied, appointments are fairly routine, with other members of the team taking over much of the treatment under the direction of the orthodontist. (I check all patients at each appointment to evaluate their progress, reassure and motivate them, and make any decisions that need to be made.) As the end of treatment nears, the orthodontist steps back in to fine-tune any adjustments and bring treatment to a smooth close.

IT TAKES COMMITMENT TO MAKE AN ORTHODONTIST

According to the American Dental Association (ADA), "a specialty is an area of dentistry that has been formally recognized by the ADA as meeting the specified requirements for recognition of Dental Specialists."[2] The ADA officially recognizes nine fields as dental specialties. Of these nine, orthodontics and dentofacial orthopedics are defined as a "specialty that includes the diagnosis, prevention, interception, and correction of malocclusion, as well as neuromuscular and skeletal

---

2   "Dental Specialties," American Dental Association, accessed May 24, 2018, https://www.ada.org/en/education-careers/careers-in-dentistry/dental-specialties.

abnormalities of the developing or mature orofacial structures."[3]

Orthodontists and their teams provide treatment of misaligned teeth and jaws through the use of various types of orthodontic appliances and techniques.

As I mentioned in the introduction, dentists undergo four years of undergraduate studies, earning a degree that is often related to biology or medicine. Before entering dental school, I earned a bachelor's degree in microbiology, which plays a role in dentistry. Having that in-depth science background made dental school a little easier for me.

Graduation with a four-year college degree is followed by four more years of dental school. Many dental schools begin hands-on patient care as part of the training in the third year. I was in a more progressive program at the Medical College of Georgia, which had us seeing patients as early as the second half of my first year. So, I've been treating patients since 1988.

If dentists choose to move forward with a specialty, they must invest in another two to three years of training, depending on the program. Typically, only the best of the best are offered positions in a residency program. I was top of my class during all four years of dental school, but I still had to apply to and be accepted into a program.

Applicants undergo a stringent interview process because the profession wants motivated people who are going to study hard, can problem-solve, and enjoy working with people.

A residency consists of studying under professors—many of whom work as practicing orthodontists—and providing care to patients through the school's clinic. That hands-on patient care begins on the first day.

Orthodontics is very different from dentistry: different terminol-

3   "Specialty Definitions," American Dental Association, accessed May 24, 2018, https://www.ada.org/en/education-careers/careers-in-dentistry/dental-specialties/specialty-definitions.

ogy, different equipment, and different tools. There is no way dentists can reach a level of training on their own or through weekend, hotel-based courses without going through such a university-based residency program. Many programs also have their orthodontic residents collaborate with other dental specialists so that they may learn about advanced treatment options.

The key point to remember is this: All orthodontists are dentists, but not all dentists are orthodontists. According to the AAO, only 6 percent of dentists are orthodontists. Just as in other areas of medicine, every surgeon is a doctor, but not all doctors are surgeons. And when you need medical care, you go to the doctor who can best provide it, right? It's the same with dentistry and orthodontics.

AN EVER-CHANGING FIELD

Orthodontics is an ever-changing field. Technologies are a big part of what's making treatment today faster, friendlier, and more efficient—just a better experience overall. From diagnostics to planning to treatment, technology is improving the care orthodontists can offer and helping us transform people's lives.

As an early adopter for various companies, my practice often has opportunities to try technologies before other practices. With each, we evaluate the value of the technology against the patient experience—we want to use whatever works best for the patient and is good for the practice. Technology can be expensive, and while it can improve the level of care, it can also impact fees. But weighed against the costs of living with unattractive or unhealthy teeth, orthodontics is an investment that has great value for the long-term.

CHAPTER TWO

The Value of Your Investment

Orthodontic treatment is a journey to better oral health, increased confidence, and better personal and professional opportunities. It's an investment in yourself and your future. Unlike a car or even a house, a healthy smile is an asset that should last the rest of your life. Given the positive impact it can have in your career, relationships, and health, it's important to trust your care to someone with the appropriate skills, knowledge, and experience. Why settle for anything less? In fact, why settle for anything less than the best?

Look at it this way: You love your family physician, whom you see every year and whose recommendations and treatment you trust, right? But what if your family physician said that you needed heart surgery? What would you do if your family physician offered to perform an elective plastic surgical procedure? Would you trust that physician to perform either of these procedures? Of course not.

It's no different when it comes to your oral health. There are different levels of training and expertise in the dental field, and that leads to different results.

Regan, for instance, came to us because she was unhappy with recently completed orthodontic treatment that was done by her dentist. But she didn't realize he was not an orthodontist until the treatment was nearly complete. During my assessment, she told me that she felt her teeth looked worse after the treatment. I did not have her records, but according to her descriptions, her lower teeth were now straighter, but her upper teeth were more spaced out and nearly hidden by her upper lip, and her upper and lower front teeth were leaning forward too much.

My suspicions of her situation were confirmed by an examination: Over time, her lower jaw had grown farther forward on the left, causing what's known as an asymmetric Class III bite, causing her lower midline to shift to the right about three millimeters. As often happens with Class III bites, the body tries to compensate by crowding and misaligning the lower teeth so they can still fit within the arch form of the top teeth. Her upper teeth were probably pretty straight before treatment, but now were gapped. Correcting that takes far more than just straightening the teeth with braces. And trying to do so without taking everything into consideration results in front teeth tipped so far forward that they become very prominent, as confirmed by her cephalometric x-ray.

Making teeth straight is the easy part. Correcting the bite and managing the side effects orthodontic treatment can produce when not planned properly and carefully monitored along the way is where the expertise of an orthodontic specialist comes in. Regan had several key issues that the treating doctor either missed, did not anticipate as problem causers, or had no idea how to address. The dentist was no doubt well-meaning, but he didn't know what he didn't know—and the results were appalling.

I came up with a plan to camouflage her Class III bite, align her teeth, close her upper spaces, reduce the prominence of her front teeth, and create a beautiful smile line by bringing her front teeth down to match the curve of her lower lip when she smiled. All in less time than the previous treatment had taken.

Again, it's not the appliances that straighten teeth; it's the guy behind those tools and techniques that determines the outcome. The training and experience of the doctor determines the movements of the teeth. In other words, stick with a certified orthodontic specialist who does braces all the time, rather than someone who just dabbles in it. And when choosing an orthodontist, choose one with ample experience and a great reputation. That can mean a better result and a more pleasant experience along the way including shorter visits, less discomfort, and less frustration.

STILL, IT'S A TEAM EFFORT

While orthodontists undergo extra, specialized training beyond dental school, and then spend their days using their training and skills to treat patients in orthodontic care, they sometimes rely on other doctors to provide additional care to their patients.

The ADA actually recognizes nine fields as dental specialties. Here are some of the other providers we use and their vital roles in helping make sure our patients get comprehensive care.

- General dentists perform cleanings, fillings, crowns, bridges, and much more. They monitor overall oral health and seek assistance for the more advanced procedures.

- Endodontists primarily perform root canals to help save teeth from extraction when the pulp becomes diseased.

- Oral and maxillofacial surgeons perform procedures such as extractions, implants, and jaw alignment surgery.

They specialize in treating issues impacting the hard and soft tissues of the jaws, face, head, and neck.

- Periodontists deal with diseases or conditions that affect the tissues of the mouth which support the teeth. Moving teeth requires healthy gums, so some patients with issues such as gum disease or bone damage that threatens the loss of a tooth will work with a periodontist before getting braces.

When needed, we also sometimes work with TMJ and sleep therapy specialists who refer patients to us. Although not a specialty recognized by the ADA, these are often dentists or orthodontists who have chosen to focus on those areas. I'll talk about this more in chapter ten.

Why does it matter who provides care? Because, again, training and experience make all the difference. Different specialists focus on different areas of oral health. They spend all day working with patients dealing with those issues under their area of expertise. So it matters who is providing your care depending on the issue you're dealing with. Again, the doctor behind the tools determines the outcome.

Carolyn is a good example of how working with other providers helps ensure a smooth transition in patient care. Carolyn was forty-three when she came in to us, wanting a gap in her front teeth corrected. She had already had braces as a child and had worn a lingual retainer ever since (a lingual retainer is bonded to the back of the front teeth). However, even though she had good oral health overall, visiting her dentist regularly and keeping her teeth clean with regular care on her own, she had lost several teeth over the years. She didn't complain of jaw joint pain (a symptom of TMJ, which I'll discuss in chapter ten), but she did have a family history of narrow upper jaw, which caused her bite to be misaligned: her upper and lower teeth didn't meet when she bit down. And her front teeth were flared far more than they should have been to have that dazzling finish I discussed in chapter one.

X-rays showed that she had the bone structure to support orthodontic treatment with braces, but her treatment also required a coordinated effort between my office, a periodontist, an oral surgeon, and a general dentist. Once each doctor had examined the patient, we met together to come up with a treatment plan, which she agreed to. Her plan included extracting some teeth that were hopelessly diseased, using braces to align teeth and create space for implants, placing the implants, placing temporary crowns on those implants to use for anchoring orthodontic brackets, and then using braces to move everything into place. When her orthodontic treatment was done, she had permanent crowns placed on her implants along with some cosmetic bonding of her front teeth. We then placed new bonded lingual retainers and also gave her clear, molded retainers to hold everything in place for the long term.

By working with other oral specialists, we were able to better predict Carolyn's results. All the doctors played an important role by maximizing their areas of expertise, and together, we were able to give Carolyn her smile back—and she was ecstatic about the result.

Part of the reason for collaboration is to ensure a smooth transition in care. But it also lets us educate other providers about what we do: we want those other providers to know where to send patients whose problems are outside their scope of experience and expertise, and we want those connections so that we can do the same. By meeting with other providers and sharing knowledge, we're able to continually improve patient care across the industry.

SHOPPING FOR A PROVIDER

Since the Great Recession of the late-2000s, we've found that some people shop around for orthodontic treatment. Rather than going to someone highly recommended by their dentist or a friend, they'll actually make appointments with several doctors for an evaluation. Unfortunately, too often, that leads to choosing a provider based on cost alone. Instead of looking at all the factors that go into treatment, parents, sometimes, will go with the cheapest provider for their children's orthodontic care, only to realize after a few visits that, as the saying goes, you get what you pay for. Every visit, they sit in the waiting room for an hour before being seen for an appointment that takes longer than it should. Their children always seem to be in pain. The assistants in the office are not trained, so the children get repeatedly poked and prodded, and procedures are not completed correctly. The children are yelled at for not brushing their teeth (instead of being encouraged and instructed in how to do better). And the treatment continues way longer than it should.

That's the type of care often found in practices that are owned and operated by big corporations and faceless investors, ownership that is often hidden. Corporate practices typically have a revolving door of doctors and team members who are overworked and dissatisfied with their work environment. That adversely affects patient care because there is no continuity, treatment takes longer, and results are not optimal. The doctors working in these environments are often inexperienced, recent graduates trying to work off student loan debt and then move on, or they are practitioners who opted out of private practice.

> *"Price* is what you pay. *Value* is what you get."
> —Warren Buffet

Doctors who own a practice tend to be in it for the long haul. They are more involved in providing care and have a vested interest in your experience, satisfaction, and treatment outcome.

Sometimes potential patients confuse *price* with *value* and feel that paying the lowest fee for a service is a good deal. They fail to realize that a lower fee is often a reflection of lower value. As part of the health care industry, fees (or price) for orthodontics are set by individual doctors offering their services. Since all doctors know the value of their treatment, they set their fees accordingly. In contrast to a product or commodity, such as a pair of running shoes or a tube of lipstick, for which prices are relatively fixed, based on the cost to produce and sell that item, fees for orthodontic services are based more on the value you are likely to perceive and receive from the doctor. That value can be based on a number of factors, as you will see throughout this book. And typically, the better value is not found with the provider charging the lower fee. The experience, treatment outcome, and level of service you receive in one practice versus another can vary widely. When looking at options in care providers you must see if you are comparing apples to apples.

> Since all doctors know the value of their treatment, they set their fees accordingly.

In the end, it costs patients who choose a low-fee office a lot of money, time, and discomfort to "save" a few bucks—even more so if the work has to be redone. I liken it to leaping out of a plane and only discovering then that your choice of parachutes was a mistake. At that point, you're already committed and if the parachute doesn't work, you're toast.

Don't settle or base your decision strictly on the fee. As you will see later in the book, we are able to make even the best care affordable. When you choose a practice based on factors such as orthodontist experience, friendly staff, technologies, and overall environment, there's no reason to dread treatment today. Our patients really enjoy coming in for treatment for a number of reasons that I'll explain in the next chapter.

Seeking multiple opinions can also lead to a lot of confusion because doctors often recommend different treatment plans. That doesn't necessarily mean that one is right and another is wrong. Training, background, and experience vary, leading to different opinions and recommendations. There is often more than one way to treat a case successfully and with similar results. In most cases, the initial visit is for an assessment and is not a full treatment planning session. The findings and recommendations are only preliminary. A complete diagnosis is best done with full diagnostic records, when the doctor has time to develop a treatment plan.

MAIL ORDER, DO-IT-YOURSELF BRACES

Too often, young adults are looking for a fast, cheap solution to fix crooked teeth. But when it comes to moving teeth, a quick fix is usually not the best fix and the Internet is not your friend when it comes to do-it-yourself options.

Take the online videos that show how to close a gap in front teeth with a little rubber band. The problem with that gimmick is that the rubber band rides up under the gums and, as it contracts, it slides up the roots of the teeth. Up, up, up it goes and before the wearers know it, the band has caused problems in the bone that holds the teeth. Ultimately, they end up losing their front teeth. Now the fix is far costlier than a couple of rubber bands.

Then there are companies selling do-it-yourself plastic aligners shipped directly to you. These companies claim there is no need for an orthodontist and that their aligners will deliver the same result for a fraction of the cost. Nothing could be further from the truth. First, they send you the material to create a mold of your mouth that you send to them. Not only is it challenging for a novice to make high quality molds, but can you imagine gagging yourself with that goopy impression material? Then, they ship back to you a series of clear aligners.

But moving teeth is complicated. A lot of problems can arise in moving teeth without a specialist's supervision. For instance, when there's not enough room in the mouth, other teeth can and do shift to make room for those that you are trying to move. Without direct supervision by a qualified and experienced professional overseeing the growth of new bone to accommodate shifting teeth, it's even possible to move teeth right out of the bone. You could end up creating more damage than you started with. That's why do-it-yourself aligners fail. The lab technicians creating the computer models don't understand the nuances of each case. With continual eyes-on monitoring by a qualified professional, the treatment plan can be altered when needed, and the end result is certain to be much better.

Again, orthodontists are trained and hands-on medical professionals who understand what it means to move teeth in bone. Remember that understanding the biology of the human body is part of our training. We spend years learning about it and we know that there is more to moving teeth than just inserting a piece of plastic shaped like your teeth in your mouth or even following computerized lab recommendations when experience tells us otherwise.

THE COST OF ORTHODONTICS— IT'S ABOUT VALUE

The cost of orthodontics goes far beyond dollars and cents. It's about the value. My goal is always to provide the best treatment possible and a great experience and make it affordable for any family budget by being unusually flexible with payment arrangements. I don't want finances getting in the way of having treatment.

Thanks to ongoing advances in the industry, technologies have improved the overall experience of getting braces, and yet costs have not increased over time when compared to inflation and other health care. In fact, compared to the price of other goods and services, orthodontics has remained far more affordable. Consider these:

- In 1978, a movie ticket cost $1. Today, it's $10 or more to see a first-run show.[4]

- In the mid-1970s, a pound of coffee cost around $1.40. Today, a pound of coffee averages $6.00.[5]

- A preowned Volkswagen in 1979 cost $5,000. You could, literally, buy a used car back in the late 1970s for around the same price as basic orthodontic treatment today.

According to CNN Money, with inflation, the average cost of braces in 1960 (around $2,000), should be nearly $16,000 today.[6] Yet the Oral B website reports that the cost of braces can range from $3,000 to $8,000 depending on the condition of your teeth, your mouth, the type of technologies used, and the length of treatment.[7] For instance, with our in-house technologies such as digital scanning, computer modeling, and 3-D printing, we can save some patients needing only minor or moderate adjustments thousands of dollars by creating a limited set of custom aligners at a fraction of the cost of full braces.

---

4   "The History of What Things Cost in America: 1776 to Today," 24/7 Wall Street, September 16, 2010, accessed May 24, 2018, https://247wallst.com/investing/2010/09/16/the-history-of-what-things-cost-in-america-1776-to-today/3/.

5   Ibid.

6   "Inflation: How Much It Costs—Then and Now," CNN Money calculators, accessed May 24, 2018, money.cnn.com/calculator/pf/inflation-adjustment/.

7   "How Much Do Braces Cost?" Oral-B corporate site, accessed May 24, 2018, https://oralb.com/en-us/oral-health/life-stages/braces/how-much-do-braces-cost.

Paying for braces is relatively easy and it always has been. Most orthodontists allow patients to pay for treatment over the expected length of treatment, or even longer. That makes it more affordable and payment plans can be customized to fit the family budget, usually with no interest. I'll talk more about payment plans in chapter four.

What goes into the equation of how much braces cost is where the true value lies. Yes, experience, quality treatment, qualified staff, and better technology cost a little more, but in the end, the outcomes speak for themselves.

In its purest sense, a smile is a reflection of happiness. It can change outcomes both personally and professionally. To put a value on a smile, on a transformation, on a lifelong boost to someone's confidence, is difficult to quantify. As an orthodontist, I've seen thousands of transformations. What's that worth? To me, it's priceless.

WHAT IS YOUR ORAL HEALTH WORTH TO YOU?

What it all comes down to is value. What is it worth for you or your loved one to greet the world with a beautiful smile?

Do you have time to deal with broken appliances because you went with an orthodontist who uses cheaper brackets or inferior bonding cement? Are you comfortable paying for treatment in an office that doesn't have certified assistants, which shows in their confidence and efficiency in treatment?

Would you compromise the quality of a parachute if you won't know you have done so until it is too late?

Value is not just the final result; it's also the experience along the way. There will always be people who say they can do it cheaper, but at what cost?

CHAPTER THREE

What to Look for in an Orthodontist

All orthodontists are not created equal. Finding the right orthodontist is an important decision. You need to know what to expect in treatment. After all, you will be under the orthodontist's care for some time (up to two years for some people), and the treatment is geared toward creating something you'll face the world with every day: an amazing smile.

But orthodontics is so much more than just braces. The braces themselves are only part of the journey. It's also important to consider the quality of care, the relationship with the provider and team, the costs of treatment, and your expectations about the journey.

Here are some of the features to look for to find an orthodontist who will give you the best care, the results you desire, a pleasant experience, and affordable payment options.

YEARS OF SPECIALTY EXPERIENCE

Experience counts when choosing an orthodontist. That's especially important when it comes to tougher cases. And those tougher cases can be difficult to recognize early on. There are so many different scenarios of malocclusion. Some of the more challenging are only seen a few times during an orthodontist's entire career. With experience come the skills necessary to analyze and individually plan each case, which leads to shorter, more predictable treatment and the best results for routine as well as complex cases.

Orthodontists are dentists that have an additional two to three years of training in an accredited orthodontic specialty program. By the time orthodontists graduate, most have been treating patients hands-on for at least four years. And many go into practice with someone else for the first few years right out of school. That's really what it takes for orthodontists to become more comfortable with what they have to do.

I was at the top of my dental school class for all four years of my initial training, and by the time I graduated, I had already been providing hands-on patient care for more than five years and I took over an existing practice very early in my career, which gave me experience in running my own business. As I write this book, I have nearly thirty years of experience to my credit.

There is a clear difference when you're in the hands of someone who has seen as many cases as I have. I really have seen it all. Am I a better orthodontist then I was twenty, ten, or even five years ago? You bet.

AN ORTHODONTIST AND BUSINESS OWNER

Does the orthodontist also own the practice? When doctors own the practice, they are not only invested in the business financially but also ethically and mentally. The patients' best interests and the practice's reputation are always top of mind. When a doctor is employed by another entity, especially by outside investors or corporations, there is a tendency to cut corners in the level of service, materials used, and team training in order to cut costs and improve profits for the owners. In fact, these cuts are often mandated by the nondoctor owner in order to increase the bottom line. But at what expense? Continuity of care and quality of treatment can be compromised when the employee doctors change in the middle of treatment. And that can happen frequently when the doctor is not the owner. One corporate practice near me has gone through four employee doctors in five years. And the revolving door spins even faster for staff members. That can be very disheartening for patients and parents.

THE LATEST TECHNOLOGIES

One of the things I love best about being an orthodontist is seeing the continually emerging new technologies. When looking for an orthodontist, you clearly need a practice with the latest technologies.

By staying up to date with technologies, we're able to more accurately diagnose and then create a treatment plan that is customized to the individual patient. The technologies make both diagnosis and treatment more efficient and cost-effective, providing shorter, more comfortable, and even better treatment. As I write this book, these are some of the exciting, cutting-edge technologies we use in our practice to help us better diagnose and treat patients.

- Cone beam computed tomography (CBCT). This provides 3-D views of the teeth and roots, and the bones of the mouth. We have this state-of-the-art equipment in each office.

- Intraoral scanners. These scanners have a wand to create digital impressions of teeth. Goopy, gag-inducing impressions are no longer necessary in our practice.

- 3-D printers. 3-D Printers create models of teeth and

produce retainers and tooth aligners. I find this an incredibly fun part of being an orthodontist.

- **Smile design software.** By using this CAD-CAM type software, we are able to visualize how your teeth will move and even design appliances to help us do it.

- **Clear aligner therapy.** Using a series of removable, plastic trays, we are able to treat a wide variety of cases.

- **Custom lingual appliances.** Working with an outside lab, we are able to design and create custom appliances that are cemented to the back of your teeth so no one can see them.

- **Soft tissue laser.** This is used to contour gum tissue at the end of treatment, which lets us improve the smile by making the gums more aesthetic and healthier.

- **Accelerated treatment.** Today's advances include additional treatments that are intended to safely shorten treatment times. They include vibration or bone modification procedures to move teeth faster.

- **Temporary Anchorage Devices (TADs).** These are tiny anchors placed in the bone, which allow us to move teeth in a desired direction without affecting the position of other teeth.

- **On-site lab.** This lets us fabricate appliances and retainers on the same day.

Every time I'm able to bring in a new technology, we turn another corner on treatment. These technologies are part of what excite me about treating patients today, and I can't wait to see what's ahead.

TEAM MEMBERS' CERTIFICATION AND EXPERIENCE

The latest and greatest technology is only as good as the skills of the people using it. In orthodontics, assistants routinely provide a large portion of the hands-on care. The vast majority are only trained on the job by shadowing someone with a little more experience, which means they often lack the skills, experience, and knowledge to provide the highest quality of treatment. Training and certification by the Academy of Orthodontic Assisting, which is recognized world-wide and endorsed by the American Association of Orthodontists, is extremely important in helping you achieve an awesome smile. Ask to see the certificates of the assistants and inquire about their length of experience. As with doctors, assistants with the most years of experience are usually the better assistants.

ONGOING CONTINUING EDUCATION

Delivering the highest quality of care in an ever-evolving field means investing in ongoing training. In addition to certification, do the orthodontist and team keep their skills up to date with ongoing continuing education? Our team constantly receives training on the newest advances in orthodontics, which keeps them up to date and able to serve our patients best. Training is done in-house (by me and my management team), through online courses, and by traveling to meetings once or twice a year. Investing in continuing education for myself and my team is critical!

A FAMILY-LIKE CULTURE

When you visit orthodontists as you look for a best fit in a provider, follow your gut feeling for how the team works together. Are they friendly and courteous with patients—and with each other? Do they truly seem to have your best interests at heart?

When patients choose an orthodontist, they want a practice that operates as a well-oiled machine does and yet has fun and treats people with respect.

At Depew Orthodontics, our goal is to change lives—period. We have seen personalities blossom, career paths become enriched, and relationships flourish after helping our patients transform their teeth into incredible smiles. We truly feel that our patients are our family and do all we can to help them feel welcome and excited to be here with us. We pride ourselves on providing patients and family members with a warm and comfortable environment. We believe our patients are special, and we prove it every time they visit our office.

> *My thirteen-year-old asked to write this review. These are his words. "When we got our kids their braces, it was more than just getting braces, it was like joining a family. The staff are the kindest there is and talk to my kids about [their braces] and make them feel important and special. The kids enjoy all the rewards and especially the cookies after their visit is complete. They are amazing and I would recommend them to anyone!" It's amazing that an orthodontist office can inspire this level of loyalty! Thank you. —Katherine P.*

ASSISTANTS—AND FRIENDS

Some practices use what's known as a next-up system, in which assistants treat patients in order of their appointment time. This means that patients get a different assistant or clinician with every visit.

The patient manager system assigns new patients to an assistant who knows them and their case very well. They see the same assistant for almost every appointment, which helps with continuity of care, makes the patient more comfortable, and really adds to the quality of the care that the patient receives.

We use the patient manager system, and it has worked extremely well. Patients and assistants are matched based on personality and type of case. Some of my assistants are better at lingual braces, some are better at aligners, some are better with kids, and some are better with special needs patients. Using the patient manager system, patients usually see the same assistants every time they come in for treatment, and they even tend to form friendships.

Absolutely, absolutely love the entire staff at Depew Ortho-dontics. From day one, we have felt like family. Appoint-ments always run on time, and they go out of their way to be friendly and helpful. My second son will need braces soon, and I wouldn't think of taking him anywhere else. Thanks for all you do! —Letricia D.

NO REVOLVING DOORS

How long have the assistants and other staff been with the practice? In an industry known for having revolving doors, it speaks volumes to have a practice where employees actually like to come to work—and demonstrate that by sticking around for years. In a revolving-door practice, assistants stay for six months to a year—they're untrained, they're inexperienced, and they don't know their patients. I'm pleased to say that most of the members of my team have been with the practice for ten or more years. Collectively, our staff has over 120 years of experience. They like working here, and it shows in how they care for our patients.

OPTIONS FOR TREATMENT

Some practices are one-size-fits-all. The braces they offer are likely to be of poor quality, and patients are not offered any better options.

They don't offer multiples types of treatment, and they don't explain the pros and cons so patients have a choice of options based on their needs.

Orthodontists are trained to be perfectionists. Personally, I want the smile to be as perfect as possible. However, part of the orthodontist's job is to listen to patients and deliver what they want. What patients want in some cases is not the ideal, but if it's still appropriate for the patients' needs, then we'll consider delivering it. If what they want is not good for their health, of course we'll let them know that. I won't do something that feels wrong to do. I usually try to steer the patients toward what I think is the best treatment, but if they're not willing to go there, then we may need to compromise.

> *My daughter was next for braces. My son Justin had already been a patient, so of course we wouldn't go anywhere else. Dr. Depew and his staff are always fast, sweet, and very knowledgeable. If you are looking for perfection, check them out. Have a free consultation. You won't be disappointed. Best orthodontist!* —Alysse B.

HANDS-ON ORTHODONTIST

Is the doctor involved hands-on in your patent care? Does the doctor position all the brackets? Many don't; they let an unlicensed person in their office place the brackets. The two most critical areas for successful and speedy treatment are proper treatment planning and accurate bracket placement. These must be done by the doctor. Incorrectly done, either of these can lead to months or even years of extended treatment. I am a hands-on orthodontist. I create customized treatment plans for patients, place the brackets, reposition brackets midtreatment if needed, and then apply the finishing touches. It's important that the doctor makes all the critical decisions during treatment that can steer it in the right direction.

LIFETIME RETAINER PROGRAM

Once you have a beautiful smile, it's important to keep it for many, many years. Since accidents happen and retainers can easily be lost, broken, thrown away, or damaged by a pet, replacing them at full price can get costly. A lifetime retainer program can provide you with replacement retainers at a substantial savings. At Depew Orthodontics, we do things a little differently because we want you to maintain your amazing smile forever. For an upfront fee and a small copayment at the time of replacement, we replace up to four retainers per year—forever.

SMILE GUARANTEE

You may find that your teeth need a little fine-tuning down the road due to post-treatment shifting. But you shouldn't have to pay for braces all over again. We offer a Guarantee My Smile program that can put you back in standard braces for only a small monthly adjustment fee, or we can discuss fitting you with a more aesthetic option such as ceramic braces, clear aligners, or even lingual braces.

COMPLIMENTARY CUSTOMER SERVICE EXTRAS

What extras does the practice offer as a way of providing outstanding customer service? How about a Brace Bus? Our H2 Hummer Brace Bus, one of the safest vehicles on the road, picks up and drops off patients in style at more than forty schools in our service area. Since many of our parents commute quite a distance to work, the Brace Bus helps families be sure their kids are getting the care they need without anyone having to take time off of work. And did you catch that? It costs parents nothing!

We also offer an amazing rewards program with contests and positive incentives for children to do their part in achieving a great result. And both children and adults are excited to receive treats such as ice cream and cookies as they depart our office.

> *Depew Orthodontics has been wonderful. Everyone in the office is so friendly and kind. They go out of their way to make things easy and convenient. The payment options and the Brace Bus have made the process so easy.* —Kelly P.

Orthodontics is *so much more* than just braces. You will see that in the way you are treated at Depew Orthodontics. Follow-up care calls, keeping parents informed of progress, and our patient manager system (described earlier) are all extras we feel are essentials for our patients. Also key to successful treatment is the trusting relationship that is built between the patient, the orthodontist, and team.

Before beginning treatment, you should feel confident you will be comfortable and receive the best care for a prolonged period of time. To choose an orthodontist, consider all the factors I've mentioned. Some of these can be assessed by visiting the website, talking with friends about their experience, or looking at online reviews. But the best way to decide is to visit the office to meet the doctor, speak with team members, and view the features and benefits

> Remember that choosing an orthodontist is kind of like selecting a parachute: the moment you realize you've made the wrong decision, it's too late to change your mind.

of the office. By carefully choosing, you will set yourself up for a great orthodontic experience.

Remember that choosing an orthodontist is kind of like selecting a parachute: the moment you realize you've made the wrong decision, it's too late to change your mind. After all, we are talking about you or your child's health. Why settle for less?

CHAPTER FOUR

Getting Started— It's Easy

J anie was amazed at what she found on her first visit to Depew Orthodontics. She had been shopping around for an orthodontist for her child and was hoping to find an experience different from what she had found with her other providers. She wanted to feel confident that she could enjoy a good, long-term relationship with the orthodontic provider she ultimately chose.

You see, throughout Janie's life, visits to her dentist meant being hurriedly scheduled for an appointment and then sitting in a treatment room, waiting to see a provider, only to find a different face with every visit. Her own experience with orthodontics earlier in life had been pretty painful, so she was determined to find someone who understood that she didn't want the same for her child.

From the minute Janie walked into Depew Orthodontics, she felt right at home. Our office has a home-like environment, and Janie was greeted warmly at the front desk. Then a member of the care team met with her, listened to her concerns, and answered all her questions. As Janie toured the office, she found it to be a modern practice with state-of-the-art technology and yet a place where staff treats everyone as family. By the time she came to see us, she had already visited two other practices, so she was pleasantly surprised and relieved to find a place where she felt comfortable taking her child.

As I've mentioned, when it comes to getting a great smile through orthodontics, the key to successful treatment is the relationship of trust between the patient, orthodontist, and the staff providing care. We want you to feel like family because, again, our goal is to transform smiles and change lives.

That relationship begins by understanding what the practice is all about.

IT'S ALL ABOUT RELATIONSHIPS

To help you get a better sense of how much different the treatments today are from those of the past, let me share with you what it's like to be a patient of Depew Orthodontics. It really is a very exciting experience here.

The relationship with patients starts with the first phone call. When you call the office to make an appointment, an appointment coordinator gathers a bit of information, including the main reason for seeking a consultation, and how you found out about our office. The coordinator answers any unique questions, and then schedules your appointment to meet our doctor and team.

That first call is relatively brief, but it is followed up with an Internet link e-mailed to you. The link takes you to some online forms to be completed. These forms are about patient health history, insurance information, contact information, and parents' information (for minors). The health history covers everything about the patient. Why do we need to know about health issues below the neck, you might ask? Because some of these can affect what happens in the mouth. Heart, blood, or kidney ailments, for instance, may require precautions to be taken during treatment. Systemic disorders such as arthritis or eating disorders might help explain some of the signs and symptoms we see in or around the mouth and jaws. We need to know about any allergies you might have, especially to materials, chemicals, or even the gloves we might use during your care. The patient may have suffered trauma to the face or a history of gum disease; we'll need to know about those things before we begin. Epilepsy can cause convulsions and we need to know if there's a chance that can happen while a patient is in our chair, or it may alter the kind of appliance we prescribe. If someone is HIV or hepatitis positive, we want to know to ensure we're taking the proper precautions for infection control.

Sometimes people have emotional issues, which can also affect treatment. We commonly treat children who are mentally challenged and don't have good brushing habits. If that's the case, we know they probably won't do well with treatment that requires them to wear or maintain rubber bands or other appliances or auxiliaries requiring strict compliance. Understanding their limitations will help us appropriately alter our treatment goals.

We also want to know if there is a history of symptoms that might indicate a sleep disorder or a disorder of the TMJ. I'll talk more about these symptoms and disorders in chapter ten.

Having the forms filled out in advance helps the initial appointment move along once you've arrived at the practice. A welcome package of information is also mailed out. For minor patients, the package is mailed to a parent. The information in the package is designed to encourage you to go online to the website to learn more about the practice. We want you to learn about us before coming in; we want you to be completely convinced that we have the place you want to go to for treatment.

With the paperwork and a little online research done, you're ready for your first appointment.

THE SMILE ASSESSMENT

The first visit to Depew Orthodontics is known as the smile assessment, what many practices call an initial exam or consultation. The goal in that first consultation is to get a good look at what's going on with the patient's smile. In the case of young children, the purpose of the smile assessment is to give parents an idea of what's coming up down the road. We recommend that young children get their first smile assessment at age seven. I'll talk more about why and what we do for very young children in the next chapter. With adolescents and adults, the purpose of the smile assignment is to let them know what needs to be done and why.

The one-hour appointment starts at the reception desk with a greeting from a new patient coordinator or treatment coordinator, who gives a quick tour of the office. During that tour, the coordinator highlights some of what makes our team members different from those found elsewhere. For instance, you will be shown the wall where all the their certifications are posted. What's important to note is that formal training for orthodontic clinical assistants is not required in most states, Georgia included. In fact, most people are surprised to learn that in many practices in our country, orthodontic assistants have no formal training or certification because it is not required by the respective state dental boards. But it's part of what makes Depew Orthodontics stand out because it shows that we care about having the proper training and credentials. Why not? After all, these are the hands that will be caring for you and your child throughout treatment.

On the tour, you'll also be shown various rooms beyond the main reception area. These include the on-deck room where younger patients can hang out after arriving at the office. The room has amenities such as televisions and video games to keep kids occupied. There's also a separate, comfortable on-deck area for adults, with a coffee bar, armchairs, and other comforts. And there is a theater room to keep young family members occupied while their sibling receives treatment. There is also a tooth-brushing station for patients to use in getting ready for their appointment. After all, we don't want to look at dirty teeth. You'll see our clinical treatment area and how we work efficiently to provide great care for our patients. This is where the magic happens and it's often a very busy place. There is a sterilization room that helps us maintain good infection control to avoid cross contamination between patients. And we have an in-house lab where we make our own appliances and retainers to provide more efficient and effective treatment for our patients.

Our goal is to get you as comfortable as possible, as quickly as possible, so highlighting our quality of care can help you gain that level of comfort. You will appreciate our cleanliness, order, and general office atmosphere. The tour also includes introductions to some team members and a look at our state-of-the-art technologies.

To prepare for meeting the doctor, a technician takes digital photos of facial profile and symmetry, and teeth from various angles. This will help as we discuss your case or your child's case. That's followed by other imaging techniques, including a panoramic x-ray, which is a screening image that looks at any issues around the teeth including development problems, impacted teeth, whether wisdom teeth are coming in or have been extracted, and so on. A cephalometric x-ray, which images a side view of the head, helps us evaluate the growth of the jaws in relationship to each other, among other important considerations. The photos and x-rays are loaded into a computer for me to use in the rest of the evaluation.

The treatment coordinator then takes patients into an exam room to go over their health history, discuss more details, and try to understand the main reasons for the visit. The coordinator shares that information with me to help me begin to get an insight into the patient's specific needs and situation.

When I come into the exam room, I visit with the patient, and the parent (preferably both parents) if the patient is a minor, and we talk a bit about the reason for their visit. After that, I have the patient sit in the examination chair, and I delve further into specifics such as measuring the bite and evaluating its characteristics. I measure and assess things such as the overbite, overjet, facial profile and symmetry, smile aesthetics, arch width, crowding, spacing, and signs of crossbites. I also look for other things such as missing, extra, impacted, or misshaped teeth.

It's important to have an in-person examination of the mouth by an orthodontist before starting treatment because that's the only way to detect certain issues. Even with all the technologies available today, an experienced orthodontist needs to look inside the mouth and touch and feel the structures inside and out to be able to determine whether certain conditions are present. Gum disease, for instance, is one of the problems that is best evaluated initially by a visual exam. A look inside the mouth also lets the orthodontist get an idea of a person's oral hygiene skills at home. Good brushing is key to good oral health, and good oral health is critical for a good outcome with braces. It's also critical for the orthodontist to evaluate TMJ health and bite issues in person.

A visual exam of the bite is also the best way to find a person's true bite, which determines the starting point for treatment. If patients have some sort of interference in their mouth, it may cause them to subconsciously shift their teeth to the side or forward to avoid an uncomfortable collision of the teeth. Over time, that postured bite becomes habitual out of necessity, and if left undetected and untreated, the jaw can grow to become permanently off-center, no longer shifting. We commonly see this in patients with narrow upper jaws. It's important that we diagnose and treat each case from their true bite, rather than from a postured or shifted bite.

To assess this, with the patients lying back in the chair, I help them relax their lower jaw, and then I open and close their jaw like a door. That action lets me hinge the jaw open and closed to see where the mouth closes. Sometimes it closes in a place that is not ideal, which lets me know their true bite and my starting point.

Once I finish the exam, I discuss my findings and potential solutions. Often, there is more than one solution, so I go over the pros and cons of each. I want to be very clear about the options available for each patient's specific treatment because, in many cases, treatment doesn't necessarily have to involve everything at once. Nor does treatment necessarily have to be done for every problem we find. As a professional, my goal is to make every patient's smile perfect. But I also have to be sensitive to each patient's desires and needs. Sometimes that means an alternative treatment approach.

If, for example, patients want a gap between their front teeth closed but prefer not to correct an overbite, we may do that as long as the overbite isn't causing other health problems.

Depending on the patients' issue, there may be several options available to tailor the treatment to their needs, including several types of braces—metal, ceramic, and lingual—and clear aligners. I'll discuss these choices in chapter eight.

Whatever the choice, I take the time to answer any questions. To help with understanding, I use the patients' own photos to explain their specific situation, and I use animated video tools to explain treatment options and what the patients may expect from their treatment. I may even share images of similar cases, showing before-and-after photos of patients' treatment and results. My goal is to help the patients become comfortable with what to expect in their own treatment before we begin, so I thoroughly explain what we will be doing, which I call "inform before you perform." We hear all the time that patients and parents really appreciate this approach.

Today, our technologies allow us to even simulate the patient's own outcomes on the computer screen. Instead of those goopy, gag-inducing molds many other practices still use, we can take a 3-D scan of your teeth, project the outcomes that are possible from treatment, and then show them on-screen. Often, that's all it takes for someone to finally decide to proceed with treatment.

Orthodontics is not like getting a haircut. It's not simply a cosmetic procedure. It's part of the overall health of your body. In addition to addressing orthodontic concerns in the first evaluation, I also talk about everything else we find in our assessment—problems the patient didn't even know they had. That includes problems that can affect overall health, not just dental appearance. A misaligned bite, impacted teeth, or missing teeth can lead to bigger problems if not addressed. Through the comprehensive evaluation, I have even discovered life-threatening health problems. Oral cancer, tumors, and cysts, for instance, have been detected with a visual exam of the mouth and confirmed with x-rays or a 3-D cone beam CT. In one patient, I even found a previously undetected pituitary tumor in the base of the skull, just below the brain. It was revealed in his x-rays, which confirmed other clinical signs I noticed in him. He was referred to an oncologist for treatment, which saved his life.

LEADING EDGE TECHNOLOGY

A big part of what sets Depew Orthodontics apart is our belief in investing in modern technology. We want to stay at the forefront of advances so that we can always bring the best treatments to our patients.

Orthodontics is a field that is always improving. The following are some of the state-of-the-art technologies that we use for diagnosis and to help develop the most effective treatment plan.

Cone Beam Computed Tomography

Cone beam computed tomography (CBCT) is a type of x-ray that allows us to look at the head, neck, and oral structures in three dimensions. The very modern looking unit is mounted on an arm that rotates around the patient's head. The resulting two-dimensional images, or slices, are assembled together to provide a 3-D view of the teeth, surrounding bone, and root orientation. With three dimensions, we're able to see things that are impossible to see in conventional, two-dimensional x-rays in which a lot of the structures of the body overlap. For instance, with 3-D, we can see impacted teeth, extra teeth, cross sections of teeth and jaws, whether there is enough space to plan an implant between two teeth, and more. We can even measure airway volume when we suspect breathing issues. The CBCT has allowed me to be a better orthodontist, because I can see things I could not see before with conventional imaging. It takes the guesswork out of complex orthodontic diagnoses and is invaluable when developing a treatment plan.

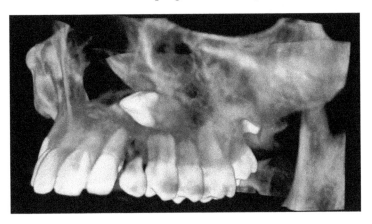

For a time, there was some concern about the amount of radiation emitted by the CBCT. But the technology has improved to where the level of radiation is so low that there is no longer a need to be concerned. The CBCT is so innovative and the radiation so low that it may, in time, replace two-dimensional x-rays.

At the diagnosis level, the CBCT helps me get a better picture of what's going on with the teeth, including those that have not yet grown in, and then better project how the teeth are going to move. With the CBCT, for instance, I can see with a cross section where an impacted tooth is in relation to other teeth. I can see whether an impacted canine tooth is crooked to the point of dissolving the root of an adjacent tooth. A situation like that alters the treatment plan. That's something I want to know about beforehand, not in the middle of treatment.

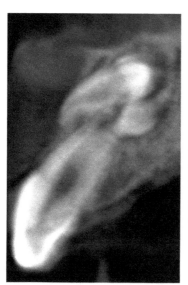

CBCT cross-section shows two extra teeth above the central incisors. One is actually upside down. It's important that these teeth be removed before they cause more damage.

There are cases in which providers who did not have a CBCT at their disposal moved an impacted canine tooth right through another tooth, causing the patient to lose a tooth. If the CBCT shows an impacted canine that needs to be surgically exposed so that I can place a bracket on it, then I want as much information as I can get about that tooth. With the CBCT information, I can tell the oral surgeon exactly where to place a button on the tooth so I have the best mechanical advantage of bringing that tooth into the mouth. By placing that button in just the right place, we can bring the tooth into the mouth in three or four months instead of prolonging treatment as long as three or four years.

At times, the CBCT may also be used midway through treatment if, for example, an implant is planned and we want to see below the gum line to ensure there is enough room between the roots of the teeth. In the imaging software, we can accurately measure the space and even simulate placement of an implant.

So, the CBCT lets us see things that are not visible from the outside. Tooth roots, impacted teeth, bone levels, bone quality—those are the sort of thing the CBCT shows us.

3-D Diagnostic Intraoral Scanner

If you've ever had a mold made of your teeth, then you know the anguish of trying to control your gag reflex with all that goop in your mouth. Today, we have the technology to take impressions of the teeth without using dental impression material or putty. The intraoral scanner uses a wand to take digital scans of the surface (not underlying structures) of the teeth and gums. It gives us a 3-D image of those structures, which we use in treatment planning.

The 3-D images can actually be manipulated, allowing us to move the teeth on the computer screen so that our patients can visualize how their teeth may look when we finish treatment. It's also very helpful for assessing the feasibility of alternate plans. The digital scan also provides us the ability to make models on one of our 3-D printers to use in making appliances for minor tooth alignment or for retainers when treatment is complete. I'll discuss this further later in the book.

The intraoral scanner has made appointments more comfortable for the patients. Plus, it's fun! It's really cool to see a 3-D image of your mouth and be able to move and change it on the computer screen.

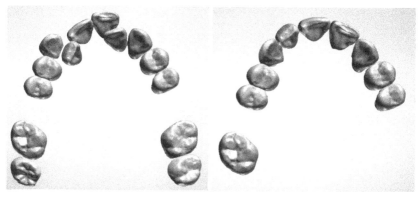

UPPER, BEFORE   UPPER, AFTER

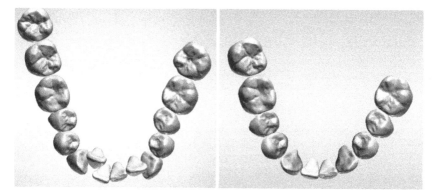

LOWER, BEFORE   LOWER, AFTER

Digital Panoramic X-Ray

Using low-dose technology, the panoramic x-ray is used to evaluate the mouth, surrounding tissues, and bones including the maxillary sinuses. The pano, as it's called, is not detailed enough to detect small cavities and is instead used to let us look at development of the jawbones, wisdom teeth, alignment of roots, and other structures of the mouth. It also helps us evaluate missing teeth, developing teeth, bone structure, impacted teeth, and the position of teeth.

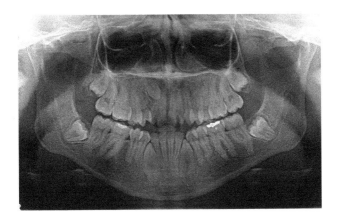

Digital Cephalometric X-Ray

Often referred to as a ceph, this is used to evaluate the growth of the jaws and determine how the position of the teeth and jawbones affect the profile and facial appearance. The ceph is taken from a side view, known as a lateral cephalometric x-ray. We use measurements from the ceph to help in planning how the jaws will change, whether through growth, treatment, or surgical manipulation. It is also a safe, low-dose technology.

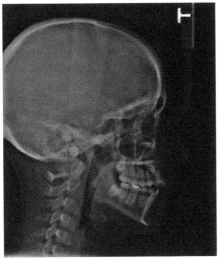

This is the standard for dental and orthodontic photographs. We use it to take high-quality, front- and side-view images of the teeth and face at rest and while smiling. We also take occlusal views—views of the biting surfaces of the teeth using a mirror—which you yourself can never see. Digital photography allows images to be instantly uploaded to our secure, cloud-based server and viewed individually or as a group. This is important as we review malocclusions or bite with the patient—or patient's parent—at the time of the exam. Since the resulting images are stored on a secure cloud, I can easily retrieve, view, and print them at any time, no matter where I am. They are also easily integrated into printed or electronic communication with patients and referring doctors.

Technology also allows us to deliver efficient, cost-effective, non-invasive treatment. In chapters five through eight, I'll share with you more details about the various treatments available today.

AFFORDABLE FOR ANYONE

Once the evaluation is complete, and I've discussed the diagnosis and treatment options with the patient and/or a parent, then in many cases, we can move forward with treatment right away. That is why we highly recommend that both parents and any other decision makers be present during the initial appointment. Some of the more complex cases require a little more planning, and for those, we may spend another week or two evaluating records and planning the case before moving forward. But in many cases, we can place brackets that same day. That's the benefit of the technologies we offer, combined with years of experience in treating patients.

Before we begin, a treatment coordinator sits down to discuss payment options. When the responsible party approves, a child patient goes to the clinic to get treatment started while the details of financing are finalized with the parents. Adult patients can still begin treatment the same day when feasible.

Through a financing affiliate, we can offer incredible flexibility when it comes to payment options. We want to make treatments fit any family's budget. Choices include initial investment, monthly payment, and length of payment based on a patient's situation and monthly budget. And the fees are all-inclusive; we don't charge for putting braces on, taking them off, and every visit in between. Our fees include:

- Initial consultation

- Complete orthodontic records

- Customized treatment plan

- Placement of orthodontic appliances (braces)

- Treatment visits

- Reasonable comfort and repair visits

- One set of retainers

- One year of retention visits

Many patients pay for the whole treatment upfront in order to receive a discount for doing so. Others pay a large amount upfront to decrease their monthly payments. Some patients choose to complete their payments during their estimated treatment time, while others extend payments past their treatment time in order to lower monthly payments, with no large initial payment at all.

We work with most insurance companies and are happy to file insurance on your behalf and accept assignment as partial payment for your account to help decrease your out-of-pocket investment.

A common misconception is that you can only see an in-network orthodontist. That's simply not true. For almost all orthodontic insurance providers, you can get the same insurance benefit regardless of whether the doctor is an in-network provider or is an established and experienced doctor who does not care for the restrictions of provider networks.

Another way to pay for treatment is with a flexible spending account (FSA). These offer a significant tax advantage and can be the most powerful way to save money on your orthodontic treatment. Many employers offer FSAs, allowing you to use pretax dollars toward health care expenses, including orthodontics. With FSA accounts, you may be able to pay for the entire treatment on a tax-advantaged basis by paying over two or three years. To take advantage of your FSA, be aware of your employer's deadlines for planning for your FSA pretax contributions. That may require you to have your orthodontic exam in advance. And don't worry. We can still file your insurance along with using your FSA benefit for even greater savings.

There are also health savings accounts (HSAs) available with certain medical insurance plans. An HSA is another way to have less money out-of-pocket and be able to use pretax dollars. It works similar to an IRA in that it accumulates funds tax-free, but funds can be withdrawn to cover medical expenses without incurring any penalty.

Fees and payment plans typically work to make orthodontic care affordable for everyone. The goal is to help you understand that high-quality orthodontics is something you absolutely can afford to do for any member of the family.

Now let's look at the various ages and stages of orthodontic care. The next three chapters will discuss treatment for young children, adolescents, and adults.

CHAPTER FIVE

Treatment of Children

In line with the recommendations of the AAO, we recommend that children see an orthodontist at age seven, once their permanent front teeth begin growing in. Usually around age seven, a child will have at least two upper front teeth and four lower front teeth and the permanent first four molars have begun to grow in. This can give us a great idea of what a child has in store. Although we rarely begin treatment at this age, the goal is to begin creating a roadmap for future treatment, as needed.

No referral is needed for a child to be screened at age seven. And since many dentists are not trained to recognize orthodontic problems, they often don't refer patients for an orthodontic evaluation until problems become obvious, which is often not until the adolescent years—age eleven or later. In some cases, that's too late to resolve some of the problems of early development.

In fact, infrequently, some very limited treatment is warranted for very specific issues, even before a child is seven years old, when there are still just baby teeth in the mouth. If you notice your child bites to the side or forward, it is wise to seek the advice of an orthodontist for children as young as four to six years old, even if your dentist does not mention it.

HERE ARE SOME OF THE REASONS CHILDREN SHOULD BE SCREENED AT AGE SEVEN:

- Problems with still-developing jaws and teeth can be identified.

- Issues that may mean problems in the coming years can be headed off. Even if a child's teeth seem to be coming in straight, an orthodontist can detect these issues.

- Early treatment may mean shorter and less complicated treatments during adolescent years.

- Intervening early can correct problems created by bad habits such as thumb-sucking.

- Early intervention can better guide jaw growth and help create space for permanent teeth to erupt into the mouth in more favorable positions.

When indicated, interceptive treatment at this age can be relatively minor and can help teeth grow in better by maintaining space from early loss of teeth, creating needed space, resolving the adverse effects of habits such as thumb sucking, or keeping bites from getting worse.

Appliances used for interceptive treatment may be as simple as a Nance appliance or lingual arch. These are known as passive appliances because they don't move teeth; they hold teeth where we want them to stay. The Nance and lingual arch appliances are used to hold space for the premolars (the teeth in front of the molars) to grow in. Once the baby molars fall out, the space can close up very quickly if an appliance is not used to maintain the space. Such appliances are not critical for everybody, but some patients are so tight on space that if we can save the space with a Nance on the upper, or a lingual arch on the lower, it helps to preserve that space. They are, generally, placed in the mouth as part of an interceptive move, and left in place until full treatment starts.

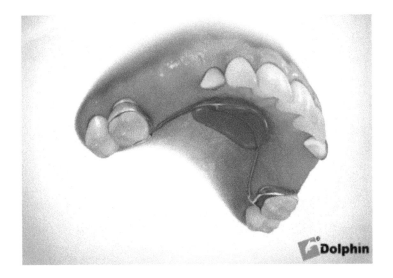

Sometimes early interception means the orthodontist refers your child back to the dentist for early removal of one or more baby teeth to avert a developing problem. It's critical to heed this advice because ignoring it can lead to detrimental problems as other teeth attempt to grow in. I call such interception "guidance of eruption."

Another limited form of interceptive treatment is a simple expander to make room for the incisors as they grow in. Interceptive treatment can also address habits such as thumb-sucking and tongue thrusting. I'll discuss this in more detail a little later in this chapter.

Full Phase I treatment is early treatment that is often recommended for children between the ages of eight and nine when all four incisors are fully erupted into the mouth. At this age, children have a mixed dentition: a combination of baby teeth and permanent teeth. The goal of Phase I treatment often involves changing the shape of the jawbones and creating space for teeth to erupt into the mouth. Sometimes this is indicated for aesthetic or social reasons. And sometimes we recommend it to avoid unnecessary trauma, which can occur with an overjet, which I'll discuss later in the chapter.

In my practice, maybe 15 percent of the youngest patients I see undergo Phase I treatment. I treat patients as I would treat my own kids, employing Phase I only if it's necessary. Parents appreciate that we don't automatically put every child in braces and expanders when we first see them.

Multiple types of appliance may be used to accomplish the goals of Phase I. If braces are used, they usually involve just the adult teeth. Since treatment goals vary, Phase I treatment may be quite short. Most orthodontists limit this phase to between six and fourteen months. Any appliances used are then removed and the patient is placed on observation. During observation, the patient is seen once or twice a year to await the eruption of the remaining permanent teeth.

The examination for young children is the same as with all patients. We start by getting the child's history and then take pictures and x-rays. I then complete a thorough exam of facial and smile aesthetics, the bite, the teeth and soft tissues of the mouth, and the jaw joints. After the exam is complete, I sit down with the parents to discuss what we found during the exam.

If Phase I treatment is recommended, we usually wait until the child is eight years old. Very rarely do we start early intervention treatment on seven-year-olds. Instead, at age seven, we give the parents a game plan and begin getting the child ready to start treatment. If there's no need for Phase I treatment, then I discuss with parents what to anticipate down the road. I continue to follow that child with appointments once or twice a year to monitor the growth and development of the teeth and jaws until it is time to begin treatment.

When we discuss Phase I treatment with patients and parents, we also discuss the probability that Phase II treatment may be needed. Phase II treatment is commonly started after the eruption of all the permanent teeth around age twelve or thirteen. I'll talk more about Phase II later in this chapter and in chapter six.

PHASE I TREATMENT

- All children should be screened at age seven.
- If Phase I treatment is recommended, it usually begins at age eight or nine.
- Earlier treatment may be needed for specific reasons.
- Treatment is typically only recommended when needed to create space or guide the growth of the jaws into the best position for permanent teeth to come in.
- Treatment typically lasts six to fourteen months.

MALOCCLUSIONS

Malocclusion is an issue that anyone can face, whether the patient is a child, teenager, or adult. Occlusion, or the bite, is the foundation of both form and function in the mouth. *Malocclusion* is Latin for a "bad bite." Malocclusions—and treatment for them—can differ in children and adults. There are three classes of bite.

Class I. A Class I bite is the ideal bite in a child or adult: the upper molars are slightly behind the lower molars. Usually there is only a slight overbite, where the front teeth overlap the lower front teeth, and a slight overjet, where the teeth if the top jaw extends out further than the lowers. The upper back teeth are slightly behind the lower teeth so they interlock, as a gear or cogs on a wheel do.

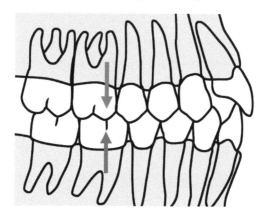

Class II. In a Class II bite, the upper molars are in front of the lower molars. That might be because the teeth grew in that way. Or it could be because of a jaw discrepancy where the upper jaw is too far forward compared to the lower jaw. Most commonly, it's because the lower jaw has not grown far enough forward. These patients typically have excessive overbite and/or overjet, sometimes referred to as buck teeth.

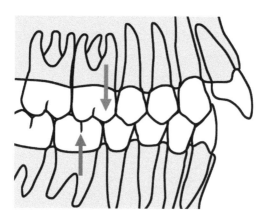

Class III. In a Class III bite, the upper molars are too far behind the lower molars. The front teeth are likely in an underbite where the lower incisors are in front of the upper incisors. This is often referred to as a bulldog look. As with a Class II bite, this is often because of a jaw size discrepancy.

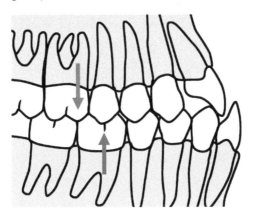

Due to the underlying hard tissues of teeth and bones, each of these bites has a typical associated profile, or facial appearance:

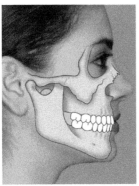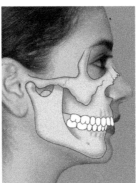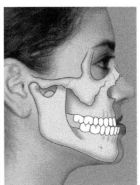

- In patients with Class I bites, the upper lip, lower lip, and chin are in line with each other, giving a balanced and pleasing profile.

- In patients with Class II bites, the lower lip and chin are recessed behind the upper lip.

- In patients with Class III bites, the lower lip and chin are in front of the upper lip.

Now let's look at other issues that we address in children.

ISSUES PHASE I ADDRESSES

Other issues that determine whether Phase I treatment is needed include the following:

Narrow Upper Jaw

A narrow upper jaw can often result in a crossbite, where all the upper back teeth rest inside the lower teeth—the opposite of how the bite should be. This is something we prefer to address with Phase I treatment. When children have a narrow upper jaw, they will experience crowding of their upper teeth. In fact, when a jaw is very narrow, the teeth may have so much trouble erupting into the mouth they may become impacted, meaning they cannot grow in properly.

Since the canines are some of the last teeth to push into the mouth, they only get whatever room is left over after all the other teeth are in. The canines are the teeth on the corners of the mouth, upper and lower, on either side of the incisors (the four teeth in the front). If there's no room left, they'll go off-path and erupt in a very unusual position. Commonly, they'll grow forward out of the gums, resulting in what gives the unattractive appearance of fangs. Almost as commonly, they'll erupt behind the row of teeth into a crossbite. And very often, they're not even able to grow into the mouth at all. They become impacted or buried under the surface of the gums in the front of the mouth or in the tissue in the roof of the mouth.

With Phase I treatment, the solution for a narrow upper jaw is to widen it using an expansion appliance. Following that, all the front teeth are moved to the center to make room for the canine teeth to naturally erupt in their place as intended. Making more room for all the teeth to grow in as they develop is much easier on the child than coming back at a later date and taking care of those impacted teeth.

There are other benefits to upper jaw expansion that are not so directly related to the teeth and bite. Expanding the jaw also decreases the chance of having to remove any permanent teeth later on. It also improves nasal breathing by opening a restricted airway, and it improves speech by making more room for the tongue to form sounds such as S and T in the roof of the mouth.

Bone expansion is easier in kids ages eight to nine. The expansion appliance works because, in the roof of the mouth, the palate, there is a suture line, the place where the bones of the head have not fused yet. Until that suture fuses during the teen years, those bones can be pushed apart quite easily with little discomfort. The suture can be stretched, and then new bone can be stimulated to grow in the suture.

Expanders can be fixed (attached) or removable. I prefer the Hyrax fixed appliance because it is better at creating true bone expansion. The fixed expander is usually anchored or bonded to the molars with bands. The parent turns the expander with a supplied key. Each turn creates a quarter millimeter of expansion. Over several weeks' time, that can mean expansion of up to eleven millimeters.

Expanding the jawbone itself, instead of moving teeth, results in more stability and a better turnout than just pushing the teeth outward. When the jawbones are widened, the teeth move along with the jaw. Pushing on the teeth with removable or more flexible fixed appliances, without moving the jawbone, can cause the teeth to flare out— that's merely a temporary fix. This concept is especially crucial when movements are done later: in teenagers, the suture is less movable than it is in children, and in adults; it is fused and considered immovable.

During treatment, I check the appliance at regular intervals to ensure it is staying in place, is being cleaned effectively, and is working properly. The appliance only widens the upper jaw. Occasionally, we use an expander on the lower jaw, but for mild changes, the lower jaw will often follow the development of the upper jaw.

We also prefer using expanders in Phase I because children adapt much more easily to having the palate expander in their mouth. They're actually excited about it, whereas teenagers often find it uncomfortable to wear.

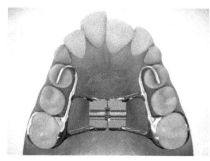
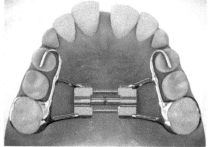

Custom made expansion appliance cemented to upper molars

After expansion, notice the space between the two front teeth

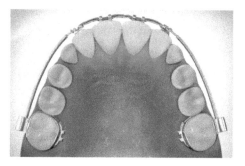

Braces are used to close the middle space and make more space for the permanent canines, as they will need more room than the primary canines

Since the expansion actually separates the right and left side of the upper jaw at the suture in the roof of the mouth, a space is typically created between the two middle front teeth. That's a good thing since, in most cases of a narrow upper jaw, there is not enough room for all the front teeth. So as we widen the jaw, we make more room to line up the teeth. After the expansion is complete, braces may be applied to align the teeth and close the space. In some cases, the braces may be delayed until Phase II of treatment.

One-Sided Crossbite

When the upper jaw is so narrow that the patient cannot bite together and chew, a crossbite often occurs. In a child, the crossbite often occurs because a baby canine tooth is interfering with the bite. As a result, the child shifts the jaw to the side to bite on the back teeth, causing a crossbite on just one side. In a child, the problem is usually postural, so we can address the situation with appliances. But that continual shifting of the jaw ends up causing it to grow off center and by the time the patient is a teen or adult, the only way to correct the problem may be through jaw surgery. This is a great example of how simple early treatment with an expander can prevent a much larger problem later on. This is one of the few problems I address quite early, in children even as young as four years old.

Severe Overjet

With a severe overjet (commonly misnamed overbite), also known as a Class II bite, the top front teeth are positioned farther forward than the lower teeth. The chin and lower lip of a person with a Class II bite are likely to be recessed compared to the upper lip because the lower jaw is too small compared to the upper. There are several reasons to address a severe overjet in a young child. One reason is to decrease the amount of work that must be done later, in Phase II treatment, during adolescence when children tend be to less cooperative. Another reason is that severe overjets are very prone to trauma: prominent front teeth can get accidentally fractured or even lost at an early age due to falls or accidents such as being hit in the mouth by a ball. Correcting an overjet can help avoid having to maintain damaged front teeth—or replace them—for life. The social aspects that kids at this age experience when they have protruding teeth and spacing are also considered. It is worth considering Phase I treatment so that the child can go through the formative early adolescent years with a nice smile.

Sometimes, if there is enough space in the upper jaw, protruding incisors on the top row of teeth can be pulled back to help reduce their prominence. Often, expanding the upper jaw helps make room to bring these teeth back and for the lower jaw to come forward. For more severe cases, a gadget such as a Herbst appliance can be added to treatment. The Herbst is a device that connects the top and bottom rows of teeth and helps hold the lower jaw in a forward position to encourage it to grow in that direction as the child develops. Overjet treatment in children is for those cases that are deemed moderate to severe. If a child comes in at age seven or eight and has relatively straight teeth with a mild to moderate overjet, then we'll likely wait and do the correction as part of full treatment when they are an adolescent.

Underbite

An underbite, also known as a Class III malocclusion, is when the lower jaw or teeth protrude farther forward than the upper. One way of treating an underbite is with elastics, which are small rubber bands that are attached to braces in different configurations depending on the situation. Treating an underbite, for example, may involve placing the elastics to help hold the lower jaw back while encouraging the upper jaw to move forward. Elastics are usually worn full-time and are changed out at least twice a day so that they're fresh and maintain their elasticity.

In rare cases, when the upper jaw is particularly small, we may also use a special headgear. A reverse headgear is worn outside the mouth and uses pads on the cheekbones, chin, or forehead as anchors to bring the upper jaw forward with strong elastics. This type of headgear works well when used in combination with an expander since the expander loosens up the sutures making the upper jaw easier to move. The headgear is worn only at night or at home; we don't ask patients to wear headgear out in public. We find most kids at this age do just fine wearing this type of headgear.

Severe Crowding

Severe crowding happens when there is a lack of space for all the teeth, which causes the teeth to rotate or turn since they're all trying to fit in. It's like trying to make room for more kids in the circle during a game of Duck-Duck-Goose. If two more kids want to join in the game, the circle must be made bigger. It's the same with teeth. Using braces with springs on them, and sometimes an expander, we can make more room. In some cases, even more space is needed for the adult incisors to grow in. So, baby teeth may need to be removed.

Deep Bite

A deep overbite is when the top front teeth, or incisors, overlap vertically more than they should. In a proper bite, the teeth should just barely overlap with the edge of the upper incisors slightly in front of and below the edge of the lower incisors. Looking at a deep bite from the front, the lower teeth are, basically, hidden by the upper teeth because of the overlap. With a deep bite, when the teeth are partly open, the front and back teeth are at different levels; from front to back, the biting surfaces of the teeth form a curve like the base of a rocking chair. A deep bite can be caused by the upper incisors erupting too far, or more commonly, when the lower incisors erupt too far. Deep bites tend to get worse with time and can lead to excessive wear on the teeth and issues with the jaw joint or chewing muscles. Even if the bite is otherwise perfect, it is important to correct a deep overbite.

There are a number of methods for correcting a deep bite including using braces and positioning them in a way to address the cause of the overbite. Some other auxiliaries can aid the braces and accelerate their effect. Depending on the cause of a deep bite, correcting it may involve moving the upper incisors up or the lower incisors down, or waiting until Phase II and moving the lower premolars up to bring all the lower teeth to the same level. Or, the correction may require a combination of all three movements.

Open Bite

Children often develop an open bite in their front teeth as a result of thumb-sucking, poor tongue-posture habits, bone growth, or an airway constriction caused by chronically swollen adenoids or tonsils. An anterior open bite, as it is known, is when there is a vertical opening between the edges of the upper and lower incisors. An open bite can tend to wear down the back teeth over time, although open bites can also occur in the back teeth.

Parents often try to address an anterior open bite in very small children with home remedies. But if those don't solve the problem, then we have habit appliances that are very effective. The appliances attach behind the front teeth and have a wire cage positioned in the palate. The cages are designed differently, depending on which type of habit is to be corrected.

The appliance to correct thumb-sucking helps eliminate the habit by reminding children to remove their thumb from their mouth when they are semiconscious since thumb-sucking is not usually a conscious act when children are wide awake. It mostly happens when they are going to sleep, watching television, or otherwise not paying attention. Some kids suck on two fingers instead of a thumb, but we can still make an appliance that acts as an obstruction to keep the fingers out of the mouth.

The tongue appliance is a cage similar to the appliance that discourages thumb-sucking. It blocks the opening of the mouth, helping to eliminate the habit of pushing the tongue through the front teeth, which is known as tongue thrust. Tongue thrust not only causes an open bite but can also affect a child's ability to swallow. In a normal swallow, the tongue raises to the roof of the mouth and then rolls back into the throat. In a tongue thruster, the tongue pushes forward during the swallow, and goes between the upper and lower front teeth. The tongue is a very strong muscle; it is actually eight muscles. And that constant force of the tongue between the front teeth can keep them from growing together, causing an open bite. Eliminating the habit by including some tongue exercises before the teeth grow, or even while the teeth are growing in, can allow them to grow all the way in together.

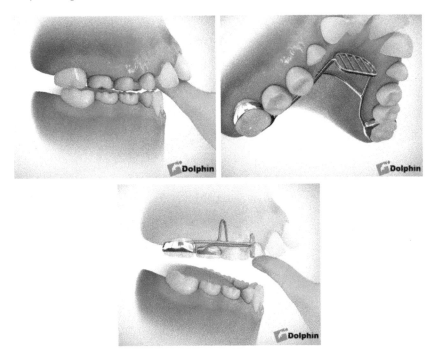

These appliances are best left in place for four to six months to ensure the habit is resolved. Once a thumb appliance, or tongue habit appliance, has done its job and the child stops this destructive habit, the teeth tend to close on their own. Some patients only need the habit appliance, they don't even need braces to close the open bite.

As with all orthodontic treatment, compliance is key to a great outcome in Phase I. Back to the saying of my professor: "Orthodontics is a specialty of dentistry in which a *professional* depends on a *juvenile* to achieve an *ideal* result." We have found in today's busy environment that we can get better results if we use treatments that do not depend so much on the patients or their parent for compliance. When determining which treatments to use in Phase I, we look at the situation as a whole. That includes taking into account the parents' availability. Parents often need to be involved in the maintenance of children's teeth during Phase I, including watching the foods they eat to avoid broken braces and helping them switch out elastics as prescribed.

Phase I treatment typically lasts around twelve months. We try to limit the time frame for Phase I treatment to keep from burning out the kids on orthodontic care. Our goal with Phase I is to achieve a lot of big goals in a short amount of time—big goals that can lay the foundation for a lifetime of better smiles.

BEYOND PHASE I

If Phase I treatment is indicated but not done, then treatment in the teen years may take considerably longer. Plus, there is a risk that some of the corrections that could have been done in Phase I will no longer be an option. For instance, impacted teeth in teenagers can do considerable damage that could have been avoided with Phase I treatment. And once the suture in the roof of the mouth is fused, surgery is often required for an adult to correct a crossbite.

Once Phase I treatment is complete, the patients wear retainers at night to maintain the improvements until they begin Phase II treatment. Basically, having two phases of treatment is taking a difficult case and dividing it into two easier parts. Instead of the patient undergoing orthodontic treatment for two and a half to three years as an adolescent or teen, the treatment is divided into two parts of fewer than eighteen months each, with the easier part being Phase II.

One of my most interesting and challenging Phase I cases was that of Camden, who came to me when she was six years old. From her panoramic x-ray, I could see that her upper incisors were likely to have trouble growing in. Her upper jaw was so narrow that there just wasn't room for all her teeth. Unfortunately, her mother rejected my advice to expand her upper jaw at that young age, before the teeth tried to grow in.

I next saw Camden at age eight. Mom was concerned that her lateral incisors had grown in, but her two central incisors had not. Her central incisors were a year late. With 3-D images taken on our cone beam CT machine, I found that not only was Camden's jaw very narrow, but she had two extra, misshaped teeth blocking the path of eruption for her two centrals. I was also able to measure on the 3-D images the size of the central incisors versus the size of the space available between the lateral incisors. There was barely room for one tooth, let alone two. That meant that, not only did Camden still need to have her jaw expanded, but two extra teeth also needed to be removed. In addition, the central incisors were pointing forward, rather than down. Treatment involved widening her upper jaw with an expander, then having an oral surgeon remove Camden's extra teeth, and also place attachments with a gold chain on the two teeth that were stuck. These were used to slowly bring her centrals down into her mouth, using braces on her other teeth for leverage. After about a year of careful traction, we were able to put brackets on the centrals and straighten them up.

Camden was excited to finally have front teeth. We then gave her retainers to wear for a few years and give her a break from orthodontic treatment. She came back as a teenager for a short course of Phase II treatment to finalize the alignment of her remaining teeth that had grown in. Today, she has a beautiful, broad smile with those two mysterious teeth proudly showing right in the middle!

While not every child will need additional treatment after Phase I, the majority of children do. Phase I treatment is largely about correcting jaw development, creating the ideal structures for the remaining teeth to erupt into the mouth. But nature is nature; even with the ideal jaw, there's no guarantee the remaining sixteen teeth will erupt perfectly straight. That's why most children who undergo Phase I treatment usually need Phase II. But the hard work is done in Phase I.

CHAPTER SIX

Treatment of Adolescents

J asmine first came to us at age thirteen. As a young child, she had a pretty smile with straight teeth. But throughout fifth and sixth grade, her teeth became more and more crooked. Peers at that age can be very cruel, and by seventh grade, Jasmine's self-esteem had suffered and she was so embarrassed by her smile that she never showed it. Even getting her to smile for our diagnostic photos was a challenge.

By the time her parents brought her in to see us, she had a narrow smile with canine or cuspid teeth that stuck out like fangs. Using SmartClip self-ligating braces, we were able to provide her with an incredible smile in just sixteen months. When her braces came off, there were big celebrations in our office and when she got home. I've never seen a happier patient. She could not quit smiling for days. She has now started school for her career in journalism and feels her new smile will take her places she wouldn't have been able to go without it.

Adolescents often have issues that are not seen in younger kids or adults. By the time children reach adolescence, most of their primary, or baby, teeth will have fallen out and have been replaced by their permanent, or adult, successors. But even when Phase I treatment aligns the jaws, the chances of all those teeth coming in perfectly straight are fairly slim. If a child does not have Phase I treatment, most of the issues can still be addressed later; it's just a little more challenging.

Treatment of adolescents is, generally, termed comprehensive, or full, treatment, since it involves correcting *all* problems in tooth alignment and jaw size. If the patient has had Phase I treatment, comprehensive care is called Phase II treatment. Phase II treatment is designed to correct any bite issues that may have developed since Phase I, to align those permanent teeth that have erupted into the mouth since Phase I, and to apply any finishing aesthetic touches. Treatment of adolescents (comprehensive and Phase II) is commonly started around age twelve or thirteen, and the treatment times and goals can vary.

As mentioned in the last chapter, Phase I is done on children usually around age eight or nine. Once that is complete, there's a small window, around ages ten and eleven, when Phase I treatment is retained and before Phase II begins. We don't usually treat adolescents during those in-between years because they have so many teeth falling out and growing in during that time. So, when children age ten to eleven come in to our office, we usually monitor them and provide interceptive treatment only if needed.

For patients who have undergone Phase I treatment, Phase II is more or less fine-tuning. Once the palate has been expanded to create room for all the teeth, aligning those teeth is much easier. But patients who have not undergone Phase I treatment may have more difficult corrections as teenagers. For instance, if the palatal expansion wasn't done as part of Phase I treatment, it can still be done in many patients up to age fourteen with minimal discomfort.

Comprehensive, or full, orthodontic treatment implies that braces are applied to all of the teeth and that the adolescent patients have all of their adult teeth. Comprehensive cases are usually more complex in nature than other types of treatment. They can involve a myriad of appliances and auxiliaries that can be used along with the braces.

Adolescents and adults are all considered to be comprehensive cases. However, the orthodontic needs of adolescents and adults vary greatly. So, for the purposes of defining the two, I will refer to comprehensive treatment as full treatment when talking about adolescents in this chapter, whether they have undergone Phase I or not. In the next chapter, I will talk about comprehensive treatment for adults.

As a parent, you may wonder why orthodontic treatment is necessary at this age when the orthodontic problems of adolescence can also be treated in adulthood. There are a couple of reasons: Problems in the mouth, left untreated, only worsen over time. A problem that can be fixed in adolescence can be more complicated—and costlier—to repair in adulthood. Plus, there is a social stigma associated with crooked teeth, something that is keenly felt at any age, but perhaps more so during the teen years. So, our goal is to have treatment completed by the time an adolescent enters high school.

Adolescent and teen treatment can be pretty terrific, all things considered. Everyone loves a great smile, and to see that created in young people just as they begin their high school years is an amazing thing. When their braces come off, I am so excited for them because I know that their smile—the smile that we created—will be with them when they do well in school, at their graduation ceremony, at their first kiss, at their first job interview, on their wedding day, when they greet their children ... It will be with them when they celebrate any event in life.

COMPREHENSIVE/PHASE II CORRECTIONS

As does Phase I, Phase II also deals with special circumstances occurring during development. Again, if not treated earlier, many of the same issues of Phase I can be addressed now. Here are some of the issues Phase II treatment addresses.

Overjet

With excessive overjet, the goal is to move the upper front teeth backwards while closing any spaces, and grow the lower jaw farther forward and harness the potential of the growth spurt during adolescence. While significant overjet is best initially addressed in Phase I, addressing a mild to moderate overjet during adolescence or early teen years is quite appropriate. This can be done with different kinds of bite correctors such as the Herbst, Motion, Mara, or Forsus appliances. Alternatively, with excellent compliance, it can be done with elastics attached to the braces.

Underbite

The goal in correcting an underbite is to slow down the lower jaw growth and make the upper jaw and teeth come forward. An underbite is something that Phase I begins to address and Phase II finishes addressing. The jaws are genetically determined to grow at a certain rate. Even if an underbite is corrected in Phase I, because of the movement of the jaws, the jaws can revert toward their former position a little bit between Phase I and Phase II since the lower jaw continues to grow faster than the upper. Taking advantage of jaw development in both phases usually corrects the bite.

Occasionally, underbites are more "dental" in origin, having little to do with jaw growth. They can occur, for example, if the upper front teeth tip back and are crowded, and the lower teeth tip forward.

Crossbite

Crossbites can be addressed in Phase I or Phase II. Crossbites often lead to crowding, impacted canine teeth, and unusual tooth wear. Crossbites can occur with the back teeth, front teeth, or even individual teeth. As a preventive measure, we prefer to address crossbites during Phase I before the canine teeth try to erupt. However, we can still correct a crossbite with expansion appliances, braces, springs, or elastics if patients don't come in for a first consult until they are an adolescent.

APPLIANCES TO CORRECT THE TEETH AND BITE

The appliances used in Phase II and comprehensive treatment are either fixed or removable. I prefer using braces along with appliances that are fixed in place. That prevents having to depend so much on patient compliance, and helps treatment go faster. Then, again, if a patient can demonstrate a great level of compliance, elastics can often be used to make some of the corrections that fixed appliances make.

Appliances are also categorized as active or passive. Active appliances are used to move teeth or reshape bone (such as an expander). Passive appliances do not actively move teeth but are used to hold tooth position, or jaw position or shape (such as a retainer).

Here are a few examples of some of the appliances we use to correct the teeth and bite.

Hyrax Expander

A hyrax is an orthopedic device used to widen the upper jaw when we need to correct a crossbite of the back teeth and make space for alignment of the front teeth. It is typically anchored to the upper molars using metal bands connected to an expansion screw positioned high in the palate. In the standard design, a parent turns the expansion screw, often daily, until the doctor is pleased with the amount of expansion. That can take several weeks or even months.

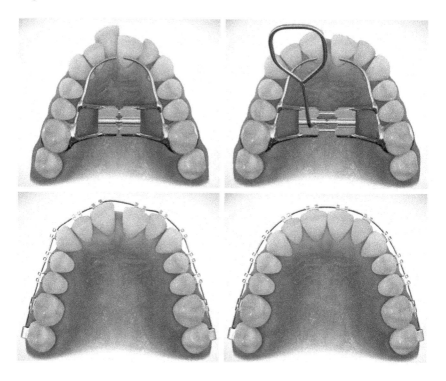

Forsus Appliance

This is made of metallic rods covered by flexible springs. It attaches to upper and lower teeth on the sides of the mouth to encourage patients to move their jaw forward and help move teeth when correcting a mild or moderate Class II bite. It is attached to the upper and lower braces and is adjusted periodically by the orthodontist. Treatment with a Forsus lasts about four to eight months, depending on the treatment plan, and is very effective. Braces are used before and after to make things as perfect as possible.

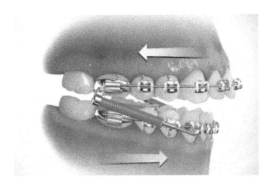

Schwartz Appliance

A Schwartz is the removable version of an expander. It is made of wire clasps, a metal expansion screw, and acrylic. This appliance can be attached to either the upper or lower back teeth, but I often use it on the lower jaw. It's a good option for slow expansion of the lower jaw.

Quad Helix

A quad is usually used in Phase I, but it can also be used in Phase II. It is used to widen the upper teeth, but it is not rigid. It is made with two bands attached to the molars and a thick wire bent into four helixes or loops. The quad helix is good for correcting crossbites, especially in younger children. It can be adjusted to turn or push individual teeth. It is usually adjusted by the doctor at each visit and cannot be adjusted by parents. It stays in place for six to twelve months and is then removed.

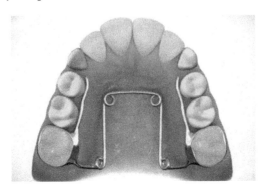

Herbst Appliance

Also used to correct a severe Class II bite, the Herbst is a little more rigid than the Forsus. It works by applying backward pressure on the upper jaw and posturing the lower in a forward position. The Herbst appliance is made with bands or crowns attached to upper and lower molars. The Herbst is usually used early in treatment and in conjunction with braces. Few adjustments are needed once the appliance is put in place and it is generally worn for the first ten to twelve months of treatment.

Distalizers

There are many different kinds of distalizers. A distalizer is used to push the upper molars backward in order to make room to align the front teeth, such as canines that are blocked from growing in properly. Once room has been made with the distalizer, braces are used to push the teeth into place.

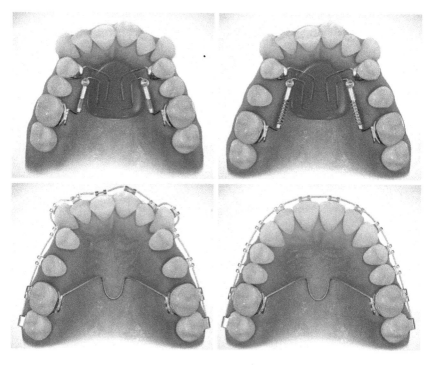

ELASTICS—A LITTLE EXTRA FORCE

Latex elastics, or rubber bands, are used as an additional force to move teeth and correct a bite. They can be attached to the braces in different configurations depending on the desired movement. Most adolescents will wear braces with colored elastics to hold the wire in place in both arches. Larger rubber bands or elastics are worn between the upper and lower teeth to apply the pressure needed to make the upper and lower arches match.

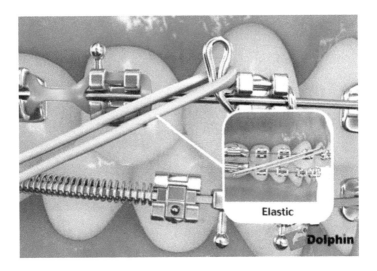

There are different configurations of rubber bands depending on the goal, such as moving a jaw forward or back.

Elastics must be worn all the time, except while eating and brushing teeth, unless prescribed otherwise. Elastics need to be changed out at least twice daily. Some patients only wear elastics at night to help hold or maintain a correction that has already been achieved.

Admittedly, elastics may make the teeth a little sore, a little like exercising for the first time in a long time. At first, unused muscles may ache a bit. But a pain reliever such as ibuprofen or acetaminophen can help alleviate the discomfort. As the patient continues to stay on course, the pain subsides—as it does when exercising—while the elastics continue to be effectual.

There are too many configurations of elastics to go into in this book, but one that is fairly common is the Class II, which attaches from the cuspids in the upper row of teeth to the lower molars at the back of the mouth. The Class II is designed to correct an overjet. Another common configuration is the triangle, sometimes called a Delta, which attaches from one tooth in one arch to two teeth in the other arch and is designed to move a single tooth toward the other two or into a position in which it aligns vertically with its opposing teeth.

Elastics are nothing to fear. They take a little getting used to and require a little bit of maintenance, just as braces do, but they are easy to wear and will quickly become part of the daily routine. How long elastics must be worn depends on how much correction is needed and the patient's participation in wearing them. A correction of two millimeters may take only a couple of months, but an eight-millimeter correction will take longer. So, the more diligent patients are in wearing their elastics, the better the treatment—and the sooner everything happens.

SPECIAL CIRCUMSTANCES

Other than the various forms of malocclusion, there are often special circumstances that are addressed during full treatment that include the following:

Impacted Teeth

When teeth are unable to grow into the mouth on their own, they are termed *impacted*. By far, the most common teeth to become impacted, other than wisdom teeth, are the upper canines. I spoke earlier in the book about the importance of expanding the palate in cases where we suspect impacted canines will develop.

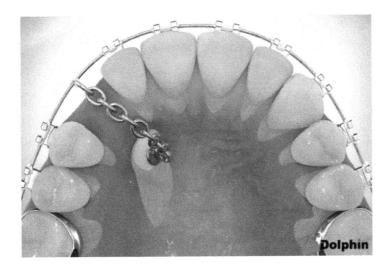

Dolphin

If Phase I treatment with expansion was not done earlier, it can be done, if needed, at the beginning of full treatment before braces are placed. Whether we expand or not, it is important to create space using the braces and/or springs to push the adjacent teeth apart. In rare cases, extractions may be needed to make room for the impacted tooth.

Dealing with an impacted tooth may require working with an oral surgeon to expose the tooth and then bond an attachment and a chain to it. The orthodontist then attaches an elastic or ligature to the tooth—or in some instances, if there is enough room, a bracket—to begin moving it in the desired direction. Remember that's what we did for Camden (at the end of chapter five) to bring in her central incisors.

Missing Teeth

Practically every day, we see new patients with missing teeth, so it is much more common than you might think. It can be one tooth, two teeth, or several teeth. The most common missing tooth is an upper lateral incisor, or the second tooth from the center, on one or both sides. Eliminating the space caused by a missing tooth can be done with a dental implant or by moving other teeth to hide the space.

If a dental implant is the option, then space must be created to ensure that the roots of the adjacent teeth are moved apart so there's enough room for the implant itself. Without something holding open the space where a tooth is missing, the adjacent teeth can tip, along with their roots. If that happens, then braces may be required again in order to straighten the roots so they are not in the way when the implant is placed. The challenge is that implants cannot be placed until the patient is an adult (at least eighteen years of age) when all facial growth is complete. In the interim, the space where the tooth is missing must be retained with a flipper, temporary implant, or fixed bridge.

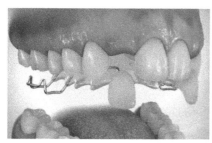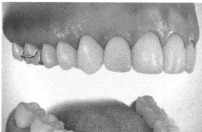

A flipper is a removable tooth or teeth. It's like a retainer with teeth embedded in gum-colored plastic that holds to the palate with suction or snaps onto other teeth. A flipper must be removed for eating and cleaning. With a temporary implant, a medical-grade "screw" is placed in the bone and then a temporary crown is placed on it. The screw can be removed when it's time to place a permanent implant. Unfortunately, as with a flipper, the temporary implants do not keep the roots of the adjacent teeth parallel, or straight. So, they are not as effective as a temporary fixed bridge, which helps keep the roots of the adjacent teeth straight up and down instead of letting them tip toward each other.

A temporary fixed bridge is my preference when it comes to holding the space in adolescent teeth for an implant later on. Unlike a conventional fixed bridge, which is held in place by crowns on adjacent teeth and requires a significant change in the shape of those teeth, a Maryland bridge is often considered temporary. It is made of porcelain and glued to the back of the adjacent teeth, making it removable after facial growth is complete and the space is ready for a dental implant. I have also developed another temporary bridge solution, which is made of plastic and bonds to the back of the adjacent teeth. Both the Maryland bridge and my plastic bridge require a little extra attention because they can break more easily than a conventional bridge, but again, a big advantage is that they do not need to be removed for eating and cleaning and do not require reducing the adjacent teeth.

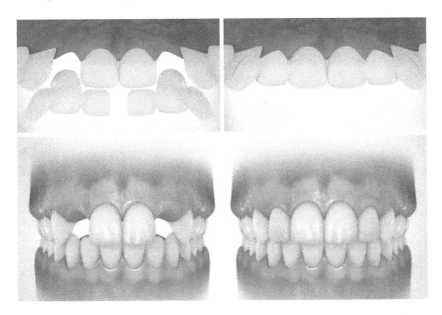

Another option for missing teeth is to close up the space by moving other teeth. When the missing tooth is the upper lateral incisor, the canine tooth and all teeth behind it must be moved forward. However, moving teeth to fill in for others can be a tricky business because it may require reshaping some teeth. Whether or not to move teeth comes down to several factors such as the size, color, and shape of the teeth. In some cases, it's a good idea. In others, it is not. For aesthetic reasons, this option is best used when canines on both sides, as opposed to just one side, are being converted to take the place of missing lateral incisors. That keeps everything looking symmetrical.

The type of bite is also an important consideration when choosing to open or close the space for a missing tooth. For example, if someone has a large overjet along with missing lateral incisors on both sides, it may be better to close the space while moving the front teeth backward, depending on the appearance of the canines. That will also improve the overjet by making it smaller.

This is where the expertise of the orthodontist is so important. When it comes to deciding on whether to fill a space or close it up, we consider the bite or how the teeth will match top and bottom, the shape of the teeth in relation to other teeth, the patient's desires, and even the gender of the patient.

Misshaped Teeth

It is common for people to have teeth that are misshaped. In females, it's more common for the upper lateral incisors to be smaller than normal or a little teepee-shaped. These are called peg lateral incisors. To fix these, we normally open a little space next to the tooth and then have a dentist use either composite material or a veneer to make the tooth the right shape and size. Trying to close the space around a peg lateral is not a good solution because a big central incisor, or front tooth, frankly looks funny next to a tiny peg tooth.

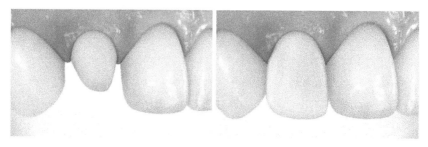

Extra Teeth

In most cases, extra teeth need to be taken out before adolescent treatment as they can prevent teeth from growing in straight or prevent us from making them straight. Those extra teeth may already have erupted into the mouth, resulting in, for instance, five upper incisors instead of the normal four. Or those extra teeth may be stuck in the bone under the gum line between the roots of other teeth or elsewhere. In most cases, we will remove extra teeth because they throw off the bite, and often, any attempts to move adjacent teeth can damage their roots if they encounter the extra teeth while moving.

As you can see, problems in the mouth can get more complicated as time goes on. Often, the problems require the help of additional providers such as dentists and oral surgeons.

Our preference is to treat patients during their adolescent years to prevent some of the complications that we see in adult teeth. While we can still do many of the same treatments on older teenagers that we can do on younger teenagers, adult treatment is a different story. For a number of reasons, adult treatment is handled differently and can often be even more challenging.

CHAPTER SEVEN

Treatment of Adults

When Jolene came to see me about treatment, she just wanted a few of her upper front teeth realigned. She had worn braces when she was younger and had faithfully worn her retainers for more than ten years after her teeth were straightened.

But after losing her retainers while on vacation, she never replaced them. That was a decade before she came to Depew Orthodontics. In that time, her teeth had begun moving back toward the skewed positions they had been in before she wore braces; they had relapsed.

We put her through a comprehensive examination that showed she had more going on than just a few crooked teeth. In fact, her adult teeth had a few years on them, and it showed: She was missing a molar (the result of a failed root canal) and had developed a crossbite in her back teeth. Her lower teeth were also crowding, she had jagged edges on most of her incisors, and her teeth were stained from years of drinking coffee, tea, and red wine.

Yes, we told her, we could realign her relapsed teeth. It would be a relatively quick treatment that would give her the results she initially desired. But what she needed, I explained, was a complete set of braces and some finishing touches with the help of her dentist to give her back a youthful smile. As with all of our patients, we wanted to be sure we addressed her wants—straightening her teeth—but we also wanted to make her aware of needs that were affecting her dental function, appearance, and even her health. Although it's challenging to meet every need and desire a patient has, in most cases, we try to address them all. That's what often shapes the treatment plan.

When it comes to adults, that plan commonly addresses the three primary concerns they have when they walk in the door: what the braces look like, how long the treatment takes, and how much the treatment costs. Since Jolene had an upcoming class reunion and cost was a factor, she chose to go with a limited plan to address her relapse and decided to forgo treatment for her crossbite. We sometimes see that in adults. They will, ultimately, choose less-than-ideal options for their own treatment. (Yet those same adults wouldn't think of skimping on treatment for their kids. They only want the best when it comes to treating their children.)

The good news for Jolene and for all our adult patients is that we love the challenges that come with treating them, and we have some great technologies—and great aesthetic options—that make adult orthodontics the best it's ever been.

MORE THAN JUST STRAIGHTENING A TOOTH

Adult orthodontic treatment can range from relatively simple treatment, moving just a few teeth, to dealing with more complex issues that require braces and other appliances. Sometimes the issues are so complex that the optimal correction requires more advanced procedures.

Many adults we see are like Jolene. They had braces as youngsters, but for one reason or another, they quit wearing their retainers and they experienced relapse. Their teeth moved back toward where they were before the braces. We also see patients who had nice, straight teeth when they were young, so they never wore braces. But over time, their teeth moved. Whether or not they wore braces in their youth, many adults look to have everything realigned and get back their smile.

We also commonly see adults who needed braces when they were young but never had the opportunity for orthodontic treatment. For one reason or another, before showing up at my practice, they also never had orthodontic treatment as an adult. Then they reach a point in their life where they're more established—they've got a stable income, the mortgage is paid off, the kids are off to college—and they decide it's time to do something for themselves. For these adults, treatment tends to be more complex. Sometimes it's far more complex because we no longer have the advantage of youthful growth on our side to help with tooth and jaw movement.

Whether it's a young adult only a few years out of braces, someone who wore braces decades earlier, or someone who needed braces but never wore them, we have different treatments to address their needs and wants.

Teeth move. They are not set in stone; they are set in bone and soft tissue, which are both quite dynamic. Over time, the body changes. Hair changes color, the face develops wrinkles, skin loses its tone—and teeth move. Adults who come in for treatment for relapsed teeth, as Jolene did, typically want to correct some mild spacing issues or move one or two teeth back into place because they want to look more attractive and youthful.

For minor issues, we have some short-term, inexpensive treatment options. For instance, treatment for minor relapse may involve wearing braces, clear aligners, or even just a retainer for a few months. Treating true relapse is comparatively easy if the bite itself has remained in its corrected state from previous braces—for instance, if a malocclusion (or bad bite) such as an overjet remains corrected, but some of the teeth have shifted and become crooked (which is what most relapse is). The key is to have the issue addressed earlier rather than later since any relapse will only worsen over time.

Beyond simple relapse cases, orthodontics for adults age twenty and above typically addresses some unique and complex issues. Not every orthodontist works on adults, because these cases tend to be more challenging, addressing issues not commonly seen in young people. With kids, we can take advantage of, and in many cases alter, their still-growing facial structures. But that growth has already occurred in adults, so treatment is often more complex.

Some of the challenging issues that are more commonly seen in adults include the following:

Worn, Cracked Teeth

Adult teeth often show the years of wear and tear. They're often worn down, meaning they're flat on the edges, and they're often shorter in length—sometimes too short. That's often the case with people who have a deep overbite. More commonly, when adults have a functional problem in their mouth, they talk, chew, and even grind their teeth in a way that, over time, causes their teeth to wear unevenly. When their teeth get straightened, the wear becomes more obvious because the edges were unevenly worn down when they were crooked.

Sometimes if the wear is minor, we can reshape the teeth a bit by rounding off the corners. Sometimes those teeth require some restoration by a dentist—composites, veneers, or crowns—to bring them back to their natural size and shape. Most permanent restorations, other than fillings to repair decayed teeth, should wait until the braces are finished since we want them to be made with the teeth in their final positions.

Missing Teeth

Missing teeth in adults are usually the result of decay, periodontal disease, or injury. Again, there are different options for dealing with missing teeth, which I discussed in the last chapter when talking about congenitally missing teeth. These often involve different providers.

In an adult, however, when a tooth has been missing for years and left uncorrected, the teeth adjacent to the space tend to drift and tip toward the space, throwing the bite off. We will often see the opposing tooth, typically an upper molar opposite a missing lower molar, move down into the space of the absent tooth making the bite even worse. In order to replace the missing tooth with a bridge or implant, not only must the bite be corrected, but the teeth next to the space must be brought upright and the opposing tooth moved back up into line. Braces are the best way to do this.

Crowns

Adults tend to have more crowns than children. Crowns are sometimes not the exact shape of a natural tooth and the material they are made of makes them more difficult to bond brackets to. So we must use special bonding techniques. Sometimes crowns need to be replaced after orthodontic treatment. When there are multiple crowns, I'll often consider using removable clear aligners instead of braces attached to the teeth.

Bridges and Implants

These are immovable. If they are to stay in place, we have to move the other teeth in the mouth to match them, rather than having the option of moving all teeth to their ideal position. Sometimes an old bridge needs to be replaced after our treatment is completed.

Periodontal Diseases

Periodontal disease involves the health of the gums and bone around the teeth. The Centers for Disease Control and Prevention estimates that half of American adults age thirty and up have periodontal disease.[8] This condition is a two-way street: gums and bone must be in good condition to undergo orthodontic treatment and teeth must be straight and the bite aligned to prevent periodontal disease.

Orthodontic treatment can exacerbate a periodontal situation because moving teeth causes an inflammatory response in the bone. Plus, gum disease is evidence of the patient's brushing and flossing practices, which is a determining factor in the types of treatment we may use. Braces can make it more difficult to brush and floss properly, so we want to make sure the problems and poor habits are addressed in advance.

Depending on the severity of the condition, we may refer the patient to a periodontist, a dentist who specializes in treating gum disease. We also have the patient continue to visit the periodontist throughout treatment to monitor the health of the gums and bone. As specialists in regenerative treatment, periodontists are also our go-to for patients who need gum grafting to build up the bone and gums to make them strong enough to handle the movement of teeth. We may also use a periodontist for extensive gum reshaping for a more aesthetic finish.

Periodontists are among the other providers we sometimes turn to for part of the treatment plan in adult cases. Those other providers include dentists for treatment such as crowns, veneers, or composite to finish everything up. And while the orthodontist may play a role in creating the space for an implant, the implants themselves are best placed by a periodontist or an oral surgeon. The crown of the implant is usually placed by a dentist. The oral surgeon may also play a bigger role, which I'll discuss later in the chapter under orthognathic treatment.

---

8   "CDC: Half of American Adults Have Periodontal Disease," American Academy of Periodontology, news release, September 4, 2012, accessed March 28, 2018, https://www.perio.org/consumer/cdc-study.htm.

Carlos was a patient we referred to a periodontist. His gums needed some attention before we could begin orthodontic treatment to address his needs and wants. He was in his early forties when he came in wanting his teeth aligned. Some were severely overlapping, in part because his teeth were so large and there just wasn't enough room in his mouth for all of them to fit. He also had some missing teeth due to previous trauma or cavities.

In my exam of his mouth, I found signs of periodontal disease. His gums were red and swollen, so I used a special instrument called a periodontal probe (or perio-probe) to measure the condition of the gums. That confirmed he had some serious issues. X-rays revealed he had less than the normal amount of bone surrounding the roots of some of his teeth. His overlapping and crowded teeth contributed significantly to his condition since their positions made it difficult to brush and floss effectively. Making them straight was imperative for the long-term health of Carlos' teeth. Still, we could not initiate treatment until his gums were healthy. Without following that rule, any orthodontic treatment could exacerbate the inflammation associated with his periodontal disease. So, I called on Dr. Wade Diab, a periodontist, or gum specialist, to work with us in planning Carlos's treatment.

Dr. Diab would address Carlos's periodontal health and help get his teeth in shape before braces were installed. After several visits over the course of a few months, Dr. Diab felt that the longevity of several of Carlos' teeth was questionable: they would likely not return to good health, nor would they withstand orthodontic treatment. After the affected teeth were removed, we used the resulting spaces to line up all the remaining teeth. So, he only needed a couple of dental implants.

I performed a diagnostic set-up from his digital models on my computer to see how everything would work together, which helped to determine that everything would fit. (His images can be found in chapter four under the 3-D diagnostic intraoral scanner discussion.) After seventeen months of treatment, he was excited to see his new smile and committed to keeping it healthy for the rest of his life.

CORRECTING THE ADULT BITE

Treatments for Class I bites in adults are similar to those in children. But with Class II and III, as I've mentioned, we don't have the advantage of jaw growth on our side. In these cases, we either provide what we call camouflage treatment, which involves correcting the dental issues while masking the skeletal issues, or we get the help of an oral surgeon to make the jaws match in order to help us correct the bite.

Correcting a crossbite in an adult is quite challenging. A crossbite is where the upper teeth are positioned on the inside of the lower teeth. A crossbite can occur in the front teeth alone, in the back teeth on one or both sides, or in all the teeth in the mouth. For adults, correcting a crossbite sometimes involves referring them to a surgeon to help loosen up the bones so we can widen the upper jaw with an expansion appliance. We can also treat an adult crossbite with rubber bands or other methods that may not be 100 percent successful, a factor we inform patients about in advance of treatment. This option is sometimes a compromise for patients who want the correction but don't want to go through jaw surgery. Alternately, we may forgo treatment on the crossbite altogether.

For problems such as deep bites in adults, we use treatments similar to those in children. Deep bites in adults are fairly easy to correct.

However, open bites in adults are extremely difficult to correct and even harder to maintain after treatment. There is a fairly high rate of rebound or return for additional treatment with open bites in adults. In many cases, we recommend an oral surgeon to help us close the open bite.

Impacted teeth in adults are likely to be more challenging and age affects the treatment decision. In a twenty-five- or thirty-year-old, I might work on an easy impaction, one that has erupted partway in the mouth and is sitting vertically in the space where it needs to go. For that kind of an impaction, we can make room, surgically expose the tooth, attach an auxiliary to the impacted tooth, and then bring it down into the mouth gradually. If the tooth is horizontal or in the palate, we'll think twice before we expose it. With impacted canines in adults, it really is a case-by-case evaluation.

ORTHOGNATHIC TREATMENT

Len, also known affectionately as Lenny, came to us in his late teens with a concern about an underbite. He was unable to get treatment when he was younger, and the bite seemed to have progressively worsened throughout his high school years. Although his teeth were relatively straight, his upper and lower teeth did not come together properly, he had difficulty eating, and he had a pronounced lower jaw. Upon examination, he had a crossbite of both his front teeth and his back teeth. I explained to him that his issues were a function not so much of tooth position, but of jaw size. His lower jaw had grown long—forward of his upper jaw. As is often the situation in Class III skeletal cases like his, the upper jaw is small not only in length, but also in height and width. We discussed how his correction would need a combination of orthodontics and jaw surgery and that I'd work closely with the best oral surgeon around to give him an amazing result.

Our timing was good, because he had finished growing, which is important in these kinds of cases. After Len visited the oral surgeon for his input, had his wisdom teeth removed, and submitted insurance preapproval, we were ready to place his braces and commence treatment. Since he was in college at the time, he chose to use Clarity ceramic braces made by 3M. They are clear and therefore less obvious.

We were able to align his teeth and have him ready for surgery in less than a year. The surgery involved moving his upper jaw forward and down slightly, while also making it wider. It also involved moving the lower jaw backward.

He came through the surgery well, although a little sore and swollen. After a few weeks of healing, we were able to continue his orthodontic care and took his braces off, revealing a great smile, just a few months later. He and his parents were very pleased—and so were we.

Orthognathic treatment is a combination of orthodontics and jaw surgery. Orthognathic surgery is required more often for adults than for children because, for adults, we don't have the option of moving the bone as it develops, as we do for children. For in-depth information on growth modification in children, refer to the Phase I discussion in chapter five and the discussions about the treatment of adolescents in chapter six.

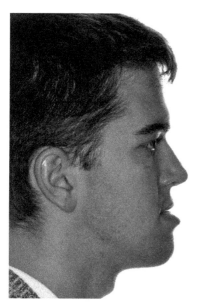 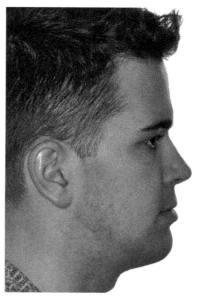

Before and after orthognathic treatment.

With orthognathic treatment, my job as the orthodontist is to line the teeth up straight, and then the surgeon's job is to make the top and bottom teeth match. That might mean bringing the lower jaw forward or moving it back. It might mean widening the upper jaw or bringing it forward. It all depends on the bite. With a Class II, for example, we bring the lower jaw forward. With a typical Class III, we bring the upper jaw forward and sometimes move the lower jaw back as well.

Orthognathic treatment requires some complex planning between me and the oral surgeon. That starts by consulting with the patients to determine whether they are orthognathic candidates, and then referring them to the surgeon for an evaluation. If a patient is determined to be a candidate, then the surgeon and I collaborate on the proposed treatment plan.

The advanced planning involves measuring, evaluating x-rays, making models, and taking photographs. The surgeon and I come up with a preliminary plan to submit to the insurance company. The surgeon's office submits the patient's preauthorization because the surgical part of the treatment is, generally, covered by major medical insurance. Without coverage, the surgical part of the treatment can be quite expensive, so it's important to determine upfront whether there is coverage and, if not, whether the patient wants to pay for it out-of-pocket.

Once we have approval, I place braces on the teeth to begin tooth movement. It usually takes anywhere from a year to eighteen months to move the teeth in preparation for surgery.

During that time, we're doing what's known as decompensation as an important goal of presurgical alignment. When the bite does not match because the jaws don't line up, the body compensates for the jaw size discrepancy over time. For example, in someone who has an underbite, the lower teeth tend to lean backward and become crowded, and the upper teeth tend to tip forward and start spacing out. That is the body's way of making it possible to chew food by getting the incisal edges closer together. To get ready for surgery, we have to undo those compensations. We have to unravel the lower teeth and tip them forward, and we have to tip the upper teeth back to close the spaces. That makes the underbite bigger than it was when we first saw the patient. Basically, we caution patients, "You'll look worse before you look better." But without making these corrections, the teeth will not fit together when the jaws are moved by the surgeon.

Once the patient is ready for surgery, new records, x-rays, molds, and photographs are taken, and the surgeon and I collaborate again to come up with the final physical plan, right down to how many millimeters to move the jaws. With the images from the CBCT 3-D scanner, we can do a virtual surgery to see how to move things and how everything will look after the procedure is done. The scans also allow us to create plastic patterns or guides for the surgeon to use to help precisely place the jaws. The last orthodontic step is to place surgical hooks on the braces to manage the jaws during surgery.

The surgery itself usually takes place in the hospital, under general anesthesia, by a team of two oral surgeons, an anesthesiologist, and a couple of surgical nurses and technicians. Generally, surgery is performed in the morning and lasts anywhere from three to five hours, depending on the complexity. The surgery is all done inside the mouth. The surgeon moves the gums out of the way a bit, sections the bone where needed and moves the jaws. Finally, the surgeon sutures the gums back in place and will often place titanium bone plates and screws (which can be kept forever!) to hold the bones while they heal. Upon waking, patients recover in the hospital with ice packs on their face. They usually spend only one night in the hospital. Then they go home to a liquid diet of supplemental drinks for a couple of weeks, progressing to a soft diet. Patients usually lose a few pounds after surgery, even though some have been known to actually blend their regular meals and then just drink them through a straw.

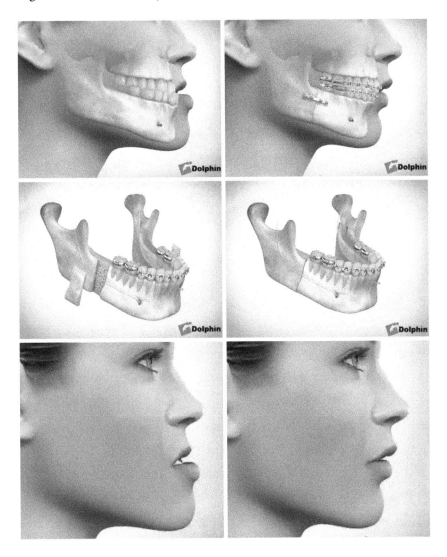

Afterward, the surgeon usually has the patient wear rubber bands from the upper teeth to the lower teeth to hold them together during recovery. Just as a fractured arm must be immobilized, the bones of the jaw must be immobilized to allow them to heal. The rubber bands also help train the jaw to maintain the new bite position.

I visit with the patients about ten days after surgery to ensure everything is going well, and the surgeon monitors the patients' healing for about six to eight weeks, communicating the patients' progress to me. Then the patients return to my care. I remove the surgical hooks, and the next six to eight months of treatment involves fine-tuning and detailing. When treatment is complete, the braces are removed and retainers are made.

One key point to note is that patients often look different to family and friends after orthognathic treatment. For instance, a jaw that protruded before surgery will no longer do so after surgery. In the hundreds of orthognathic cases I've been involved in over the years, only one patient regretted doing it. Regrets are rare because even though the patient may look different, the results are always an improvement.

TEMPORARY ANCHORAGE DEVICES

Temporary anchorage devices (TADs), or mini-implants, are a form of technology that lets us do amazing things that we could not do in the past. TADs are tiny implants that act as anchors and are placed in the bone to move teeth as specified. The concept is similar to that of headgear, elastics, and other appliances, but TADs don't require any additional cooperation by the patient to be effective.

Darrell came to us with a deep bite, severely crowded upper teeth, and moderately crowded lower teeth. He was in his mid-sixties and just felt it was time to align his teeth. The main problem was that we had to make room for his severely turned upper teeth without worsening his overjet. We decided to use a device anchored to two TADs placed in his palate as an anchor to move his molars backward. Without this proper anchorage, rather than the molars going backward, the incisors would have gone forward, making his overjet even worse.

After six months of this distalization, we were able to place a Nance appliance (see chapter five for more information and images) to hold the new position of the molars and then use braces to move his canines and premolars backward and align his front teeth. The result was so amazing that I even shocked myself!

TADs, which have threads like a screw, are usually placed by an orthodontist, but sometimes they are placed by a periodontist or oral surgeon. The gums are numbed to place the TAD, and they are commonly placed on the outside of the gums between the roots of the teeth or in the middle of the palate—wherever anchorage is needed. For example, a patient may need to have teeth moved forward but may be missing key back teeth that would normally provide anchorage. TADs give the anchorage needed to make those movements.

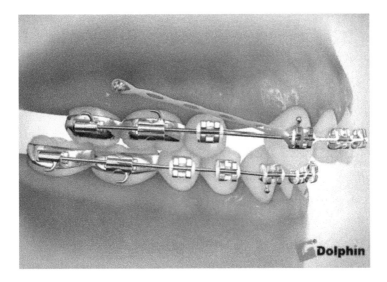

There are many different ways TADs can be used to help move teeth, limited only by the doctor's imagination and ingenuity. We can use TADs as anchor points to open space, close space, move molars up, correct asymmetries, and effect many other challenging movements.

In some cases, movement may pull directly against the TAD and in other cases they may be used indirectly. An example of indirect use is simply anchoring some teeth to the TAD so they cannot move and then using conventional mechanics to move the other teeth toward or away from the anchored teeth.

TADs allow for teeth to be moved in a desired direction without causing undesirable side effects on other teeth. While they are not needed in most cases, TADs can greatly improve the results of some treatments and can sometimes even avoid the need for jaw surgery, headgear, or dental implants. They remain in place for as long as needed, typically a few months, and are then removed without any anesthesia.

ACCELERATED TREATMENT

A question we hear every day, from both kids and adults, is: "When are my braces coming off?" Especially for adults, that can be a big concern when an event, wedding, or big presentation is on the horizon. Of all the concerns patients have, the timeline is usually the primary one.

Teeth only move at a certain rate. In fact, trying to move them too fast or with too much pressure can lead to harmful effects, such as root shortening or a phenomenon called "hyalinization," which is the bone setting up resistance to movement. That can actually prolong treatment.

Fortunately, there are many advances today that help finish cases faster. I'll also talk about some of these in the next chapter.

More importantly, the training, systems, protocols, and procedures we have in place in our offices are specifically designed to maximize our efforts at each appointment so treatment is not prolonged. Again, the qualifications and experience of the doctor behind the tools is what determines treatment. By staying on top of the treatment plan, we typically finish cases six to eight months earlier than in years past—and, according to our patients, far earlier than many of our competitors. Imagine that! Faster, better, and in a family-like atmosphere!

In recent years, there has been much research and development in what we can do to shorten treatment times by manipulating the biology of tooth movement. That has involved using different stimuli to create what is called a regional acceleratory phenomenon (RAP) effect.

The theory behind RAP methods is that cykotine molecules are released in the body when bone is stimulated to signal the cells involved in bone remodeling and repair to get busy. That's what happens when a bone is broken. The body produces cytokines in the damaged area to influence osteoblasts—bone-producing cells—and osteoclasts—bone-dissolving cells—to move into the area to do their job. I discussed this process as it applies to teeth in chapter one.

The RAP devices and methods use light, vibration, chemical injections, or minor surgical procedures to stimulate the release of cytokines.

In orthodontics, one RAP method is a minor surgical procedure that uses only a local anesthetic and creates dimples in the bone in the area of the teeth to be moved. Purposely creating these traumatic sites, known as micro-osteoperforations, triggers the repair and remodeling process. This method has been shown to be highly effective at moving teeth faster, especially stubborn teeth. One device that creates these dimples is Propel, which is, basically, a tiny drill that is inserted through the gums and into the bone a very short distance before being removed. It is used to create dimples in several areas and may be isolated around just one stubborn tooth or done all over the mouth for maximum effect.

Accelerated osteogenic orthodontics is a more invasive surgical procedure that has also been shown to dramatically reduce treatment time. This procedure is performed by a periodontist or oral surgeon because it involves directly visualizing and modifying the bone around the teeth. Since it is more invasive, it is reserved for the most extreme and specific circumstances, such as for patients who need additional bone. For these patients, grafting is done at the same time to support the expected tooth movement.

There are also noninvasive methods for accelerating treatment. Small handheld devices, such as AcceleDent or VPro5, have a mouthpiece that the patient bites into for a short duration each day. The small vibrations the devices emit induce microtrauma, an effect similar to RAP. A side benefit of these tools is that they reduce pain following appointments. The jury is still out on whether these stimulating devices actually shorten treatment time, although they do seem to work well for our patients and they definitely help to reduce pain.

Now that the treatment for children, adolescents, and adults has been explained, let's look at the types of braces available. There are many options that can help us deliver what patients need and want—whether children, adolescents, or adults—and there are pros and cons for each of these options.

CHAPTER EIGHT

Types of Braces— The Choice Is Yours

When patients come in for treatment, they usually come equipped with a few ideas in mind: speed, aesthetics, and cost. All three of these concerns can be addressed by the type of braces they choose. With the many options in braces available today, we can customize the treatment to give them what they need and want.

In the past, braces composed of metal bands wrapped around each tooth along with brackets welded to the bands were the only option for all treatment in children and adults. Their appearance came with a stigma and often nicknames ranging from "metal mouth" to "train tracks," so teens and adults dreaded the mere idea of wearing them. Take a look at the photo on the front cover of this book. Would you believe all three of these young patients of mine are wearing different kinds orthodontic appliances? Can you guess who has what? Can you even see them? Today, there are many more aesthetic options available, making that aspect of braces far more appealing.

But there are also many more options for treatment available overall. Some work better than others depending on the patient's particular needs and wants.

HOW BRACES WORK

Braces make it possible for the orthodontist and team to move teeth. Braces are a combination of several small components affixed to permanent teeth to move them as determined by a treatment plan. Combined, these components are known as a "fixed appliance," which means that they are attached to the teeth and cannot be removed by the patient. There are also removable appliances, which I'll discuss later in the chapter.

Today, brackets are placed and bonded directly to the front surface of the teeth. Each tooth gets a bracket, and brackets vary in size and shape for each tooth. These differences are dictated by the width of the tooth, the curvature of the tooth's surface, and the desired angulation of the tooth. Since today's brackets are smaller than in the past and don't take up as much surface, even metal braces aren't as obtrusive as they used to be.

The brackets have slots in which an archwire lies. The archwire goes from one side of the mouth to the other, from molar to molar in a customized, parabolic shape. The wire is the main component that applies the force needed to move teeth. Before being placed in the patient's braces, the wire starts out shaped like the arch of the patient's mouth, and it provides a track along which the teeth move. When the wire is engaged or tied into the brackets, it picks up the shape of the crooked teeth. So, initially, it looks wavy since the teeth are not aligned. But the wire has memory and as the body warms the wire up, it returns to its original shape and takes the teeth with it: in re-forming the original U shape of the arch, the teeth move and straighten.

Some types of bracket hold the wire in place with rubber bands, called elastic ligatures, which come in many colors. The wire can be held in place even tighter if a twisted steel ligature is used. Other brackets, known as self-ligating brackets, have a door or gate that holds the wire.

Putting braces on and taking them off are the longest appointments during treatment. We do a lot of work at the beginning, a lot of work at the end. Otherwise, treatment is somewhat on autopilot. Treatment is constantly ongoing. The components of your appliance are designed to constantly be moving teeth, all day, every day, with periodic monitoring and adjustments by the doctor and assistant (Remember the airplane analogy near the end of chapter one?).

When the brackets are placed, an assistant isolates the teeth with a retractor and dries them so that the glue will bond better. Then we prepare the teeth with a special chemical that etches the enamel to make it microscopically roughened. A sealant is applied to the teeth, and glue is applied to the brackets. The brackets are then placed on the teeth, and any excess glue (known as flash) is cleaned from around the brackets. We shine an LED light on the teeth to cure the glue and ensure the brackets are bonded firmly to the teeth. The wires are then inserted in the brackets, and ligatures are placed, depending on the type of bracket used. Finally, we give the patients instructions about taking care of their braces and foods to avoid, and we send them on their way with a packet that includes a toothbrush, toothpaste, floss threaders, and other self-care tools.

Treatment involves a series of wires, from small, flexible wires to thicker, stiffer wires. Each periodic adjustment appointment includes changing those wires. Adjustment appointments are also done to assess movement and make modifications, as needed, to the appliance.

In addition to the braces, we sometimes use auxiliary components. These may include elastic chains that help pull and keep teeth together, and coil springs that are used to create space between teeth—

for example, when a patient needs a tooth replaced with an implant. A more common example of use for a spring is when a canine tooth is blocked from coming into the mouth, in which case we might put a spring on the wire between the two adjacent teeth to push them apart and make more space. Once we have the space, we can attach components to the canine tooth and bring it into place.

Elastics or rubber bands also help to apply force. They are usually attached to teeth at the side of the mouth and stretched between the upper and lower jaw. They come in different orientations, depending on what we're trying to correct, whether it's an overjet, underbite, or crossbite. They're often worn throughout treatment, but especially toward the end of the treatment to provide those final movements.

If needed, a procedure known as interproximal reduction (IPR) is used to help teeth move more easily. IPR involves lightly sanding contact points to create a tiny space between teeth that are crowded. This common procedure is especially helpful when treatment involves clear aligners. Only a small amount of the thick outer enamel coat is removed.

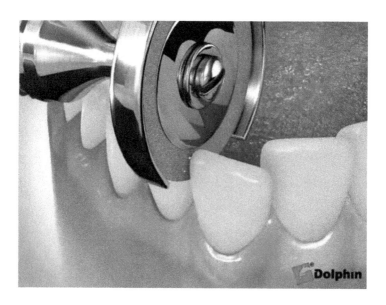

TYPES OF BRACES

Earlier in this book, I briefly discussed how teeth move with braces. To recap: Braces exert force against the crown of the tooth, and that force is distributed into the root of the tooth. The root is embedded in bone, in a sling called the periodontal ligament. When force is applied to push a tooth in one direction, cells called osteoclasts dissolve bone on the side of the tooth receiving the pressure, compressing the periodontal ligament. Those cells dissolve the bone and as those bone cells go away, the tooth moves in that direction. Then osteoblasts create new bone to fill in the void on the side from which the tooth has moved. This process, known as remodeling, takes, typically, four to six weeks to move the tooth just a small distance. Then the process begins again to move the tooth a little more, then a little more, then a little more. That's why it takes time for braces to do their job.

Now, let's look at the different types of braces involved in those movements.

Standard Metal Braces

Standard or traditional braces are made of metal, usually stainless steel these days. Standard metal braces are, generally, used for Phase I cases because we're causing simpler movements. The brackets—the components that affix to the teeth—have "wings" to which colorful rubber bands called "elastic ligatures" are attached to secure the wire that helps move the teeth. Children and some teens prefer these more visible braces because they can customize the look of them by their choice of color for the rubber bands. Each time the patient comes in for an adjustment, we can put a new color on. For instance, colors can match the patient's school colors, a favorite professional sports team, or an upcoming holiday. We often place alternating orange and black on teeth for Halloween, red and green for Christmas, pink and red for Valentine's Day, and red and blue for the Fourth of July. In our practice, we use colors as a reward for patients who take good care of their braces. If the patients don't have good hygiene, they don't get colors. It's that simple. That policy has become a motivator for good oral hygiene.

Ceramic Braces

Ceramic brackets are the most common type of "clear" braces. These brackets are either clear or opaque to help them blend in with the color of the teeth. Used for patients who want their braces to be less visible, they are preferred by high-schoolers and adults. In fact, practically all of the teens and adults in my practice who get "standard braces" choose clear brackets over metal.

A drawback of using clear braces is that they tend to be a little thicker than metal ones because they need extra strength. Also, ceramic brackets cannot handle as much force as metal brackets, which can slightly extend treatment time since we have to be a little more careful with certain kinds of movement.

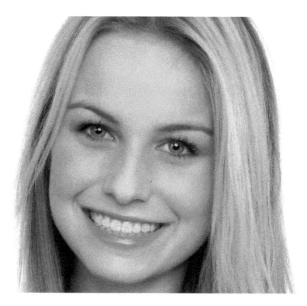

Since they are ceramic, and therefore capable of fracturing, they're not necessarily the best choice of brackets for people who play sports.

Getting hit in the mouth during a game can break a bracket and potentially harm the patient. But for most people, ceramic brackets are a great choice.

Lingual Braces

Lingual braces are bonded to the back of the teeth, so they are completely invisible. These braces have been around for many years and have been perfected in the last decade or so. They're commonly used by people who don't want anyone to know they're wearing braces—for example, salespeople, executives, newscasters, actors, and models. However, we have plenty of teachers, stay-at-home moms, tennis and soccer moms, and even a couple of construction workers who have chosen them. With lingual braces, we can treat pretty much any kind of bite.

The brand of lingual braces I use, called Incognito (3M), is custom-made for the patient through a very cool digital process so that the brackets fit exactly against the back of the teeth and the wires that go with the brackets are designed, engineered, and robotically bent in accordance with the treatment plan. Since they are made of gold, a metal that is very moldable, and they are highly customized, lingual braces tend to be a little expensive—but treatment often goes a little faster because it is built into the braces that serve the patient's specific needs.

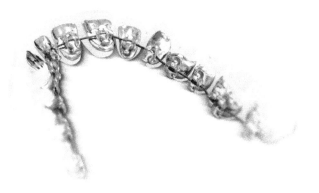

To create lingual braces, we take a digital scan of the teeth rather than a standard, gaggy impression, and we send that to the lab. There, the technician virtually moves the teeth based on my treatment plan. Then I work with the lab to ensure I agree with the positioning and any needed tweaks are done. The wires are designed to make the teeth move to that new position. Once the braces and wires are manufactured, they are sent to the orthodontist to be attached to the teeth.

Most orthodontists don't use lingual braces because of their complexity, so it's important to work with an orthodontist who has a lot of experience using them. Some claim that lingual braces don't work, but I disagree. They do work—in the right hands. And they often work even better than other braces because of the customization.

Self-Ligating Brackets

Self-ligating brackets are a type of fixed system of braces that don't hold the wire in place with rubber bands or steel ligatures around the brackets. As mentioned earlier, the wire is inserted into the bracket and a small door, clip, or gate is closed down over the wire to hold it into place. Self-ligating brackets tend to allow shorter treatment times for patients because they don't have the friction that the elastics or ligatures create, so teeth move a little faster. Think about the difference between standard and self-ligating braces as the difference between wearing boots to slide around a skating rink and wearing ice skates to glide around it. Obviously, the skates move faster. So, self-ligating brackets tend to move teeth faster. They also make for shorter appointment times since the wires can be set in place in the bracket in a matter of seconds.

Although often more expensive for the doctor to supply, self-ligating brackets require less chair time. And since they are often designed to provide less friction than brackets with elastic ligatures, teeth tend to move faster. So the extra costs are often not passed on to the patient because of the efficiencies gained by the shorter and fewer appointments involved in using them. That makes self-ligating brackets a win-win for both doctor and patient. Brand names for self-ligating brackets are SmartClip, made by 3M; Damon, made by Ormco; and In-Ovation, made GAC.

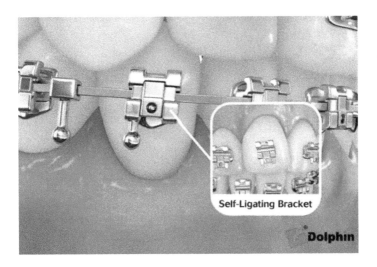

Clear Aligners

Clear plastic aligners are a technology that allows teeth to be straightened without a fixed bracket-and-wire system of braces. It's important to realize that clear aligners are not braces but, rather, an alternative to braces. However, that does not mean just anyone can effectively provide them as treatment. In the right hands, and when addressing the type of problem for which they are designed, aligners are a great option for straightening teeth. But remember that it's the painter, not the brush, that creates the work of art. The same holds true when it comes to aligners.

Two-and-a-half years before Tom arrived at my practice, his dentist had put him in a system of clear aligners to straighten his teeth. At the time, Tom was told that the treatment would only take eight months. But here he was, over two years later, still having the problems that he had originally sought treatment for.

That's because Tom's case was more challenging than his dentist was trained to deal with or even understand. Instead of a just a few crooked teeth, Tom had an underbite, a narrow palate, and a lot of crowding.

When patients are fitted for clear aligners, a digital 3-D model of their teeth is used to create the series of aligners that are traded out over time to slowly move the teeth into place. That model is sent to the lab, where a technician uses a computerized model to predict the movement of the teeth.

But Tom's dentist had followed the advice of the lab that had created the aligners. The technicians there told him that the teeth they were looking at on the computer screen could be moved to their correct position in eight months.

Now, a computer model can be a very useful tool when it is combined with a deep understanding of tooth movement that comes from years of hands-on work with patients. In challenging cases such as Tom's, getting the treatment right involves customizing the aligners to fit the patient's specific need. Orthodontists must often revise the computerized lab model, based on their knowledge of how teeth move, and then they work back and forth with the lab to ensure the aligners are going to move the teeth step-by-step, as determined by the treatment plan. Once the orthodontist approves the setup, the lab can fabricate the aligners. Combining my experience with simulation software, I'm able to predict more realistically how a patient's teeth are going to move. And it's not uncommon to go back and forth several times with the lab before an appliance is approved. That's the difference orthodontic training and experience make.

It's easy for technicians to digitally move computer images of teeth wherever they want, just as you can digitally move the image of a mountain. That doesn't mean it will happen in real life.

In the end, what Tom needed was a combination of braces and jaw surgery.

One aligner is fabricated for approximately every 0.2 millimeters of movement. That means the patients receive a series of six to sixty aligners—usually twenty-five to thirty aligners to start with—depending on how far their teeth need to move.

> It's easy for technicians to digitally move computer images of teeth wherever they want, just as you can digitally move the image of a mountain. That doesn't mean it will happen in real life.

Each aligner is worn twenty-two hours a day for one week, after which the patient switches to the next aligner. Sometimes a second or third series of aligners is created to fine-tune the position of the teeth. It's a little like golf: When golfers hit their tee shot, they drive it as far as they can. Their second shot is aimed at getting the ball from the fairway onto the green, and their third shot is intended to get the ball to go just a few feet, into the hole. Similarly, with aligners, it takes a big first series, a small second series, and sometimes, a very small third series of aligners. Every case is different, and every case is customized.

Treatment with clear aligners is largely self-managed by the patient, with periodic visits to the practice every few months to ensure everything is progressing according to plan. Since it's so patient dependent, clear aligner therapy may not be ideal for patients who have a problem with hygiene, keeping routines, or compliance.

A number of companies make clear aligners. Currently, the most recognized brand is Invisalign. With ample experience from millions of treated cases, Invisalign is likely to remain at the forefront of the industry. However, other brands are also coming into the market. Notably, 3M, the maker of the Incognito braces we use, is coming out with a top-notch product.

MAIL ORDER ALIGNERS— BUYERS BEWARE

There is a lot of advertising these days about do-it-yourself, mail-order aligners. But let me express a strong word of caution before you consider any mail order option. The slew of ads that you see online and on television are for unsupervised treatments that can have unpredictable and unhealthy outcomes. Many of the companies run well-funded marketing and TV commercial campaigns that seem convincing. But they are failing to disclose all the risks and history of poor customer service. The aligners themselves are designed by lab technicians with no to little doctor input, and there is no ongoing doctor supervision.

I and my colleagues have seen far too many cases that have failed because of the lack of proper planning and supervision. We've seen damage to gums and bone around teeth, and even the loss of some teeth, all because of this unrealistic and ill-advised method of moving teeth. I'm not just talking about a hair-coloring experience gone wrong. I'm talking about your health, your bite, your smile. With teeth, the damage is permanent.

When it comes to moving teeth—using aligners or any other form of treatment—you should go with someone who has the right training and experience and knows how to use the tools to achieve your best outcome.

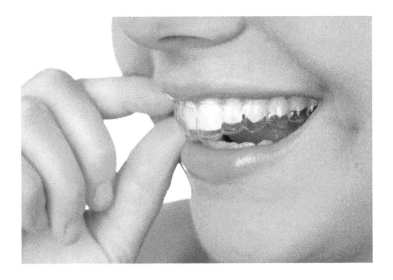

Aligners are a great alternative for people who don't want their braces to show. Aligners are removable and must be taken out before eating food and brushing the teeth. That's a plus over braces, which can be damaged by eating the wrong food, and can present a challenge to keeping the area around them clean.

For very mild cases, clear aligners can be less expensive than braces. In fact, for very short-term cases, only a few aligners are needed. With our 3-D scanning and printing technologies, we are able to handle these short-term cases in-house. That makes for a much quicker lab turnaround time and much less expense for the patient.

Added Conveniences of 3-D Printing

We are very fortunate to have in our technology arsenal state-of-the-art 3-D printers that allow for models, aligners, and retainers to be created in-house.

Progressive orthodontic practices today have 3-D scanners to allow digital impressions (goop-free molds of teeth) to be taken. From the resulting scan, we create digital records that allow us to create virtual models on the computer and virtually manipulate the teeth to simulate tooth movement. But few practices have 3-D printers that allow some appliances to be created right in the office, printing out models or appliances one layer at a time in three dimensions. We use the printer for treatment plans that require only a few aligners, rather than sending the model out to a manufacturer. That gives us more control over the aligners, makes treatment more convenient for patients, and saves patients money.

With clear aligner therapy, certain tooth movements are less predictable than they are with braces. For example, clear plastic aligners are great at moving teeth forward or backward and they're good at turning incisors, but they are not as good at moving teeth up or down or turning premolars or molars. To make treatment more predictable, we bond small, shaped pieces of tooth-colored composite to the front of the teeth in specific places. Essentially, these attachments give the aligners something to push against during treatment for increased effect.

In some cases, we'll do a hybrid orthodontic treatment (HOT), which involves using braces for a few months to get the stubborn movements out of the way, and then finishing with clear aligners. This is a great way to address the patients' concern for aesthetics, while being able to address those stubborn movements.

One of the things I like about clear aligner treatment is that it allows us to hold some teeth still while moving other teeth. With standard braces, applying force to one tooth applies equal and opposite force to other teeth, whether we want it or not. Aligners allow us to control that kind of errant movement because we can hold a group of teeth still and not get the side effects we might get with regular braces.

Again, for aligners or braces, it's always best to consult an orthodontist, one who has experience, tools, and knowledge of the treatment, who moves teeth day in and day out. Remember we are the experts. We do braces all day, every day. We don't just dabble in it. We don't rely solely on the lab to predict movements, but we work with the lab to ensure that those movements are going to produce the best results.

CARING FOR BRACES

Since fixed braces are attached to the teeth, they need extra care when eating and cleaning.

Brackets are attached to teeth with a strong bonding material, but they mustn't be bonded too strongly to be removed later, which means they can be broken off the teeth if patients are not careful about what they eat; some foods must be eaten with care, or not eaten at all, for the duration of treatment.

Food and items to avoid when wearing braces include the following:

- Sweets. Sugar feeds the bacteria that can cause cavities or white spots on teeth.

- Pencils or other objects. Chewing on pencils and other objects is a habit that is hard to overcome but can easily break braces.

- Chips, especially corn chips, work into balls that can easily bend wires and dislodge braces.

- Pizza crusts. Toppings are usually fine, but crunchy crusts can damage braces.

- Crunchy fruits and vegetables should be cut into bite-size pieces.

- Popcorn. The hard kernels cause tremendous damage to the braces, and the hulls can cause problems when caught under the gum line.

- Gum is sticky and can get caught in the braces, possibly

pulling off the brackets and wires. Chewing gum can cause wires to weaken and break.

- Caramel and taffy can cause similar problems to those caused by chewing gum—but worse.

- Hard candy, especially Jolly Ranchers, should always be avoided.

- Ice bends wires and knocks off braces just as if you were eating rocks. The extreme cold can also crack the bonding cement. Ice is often referred to as orthodontic enemy number one.

Broken brackets, bands, or wires are not only time-consuming problems and aggravating to repair but slow down the progress of treatment—sometimes for months if the bracket is not bonded back to the tooth right away.

Eating right to promote tooth movement is also important. Since orthodontics changes the bone, we want to make sure patients eat a balanced diet that includes calcium, proteins, and plenty of vitamins.

Cleaning is also important. Braces create little nooks and crannies where plaque can accumulate and be harder to remove, so it's important to spend more time brushing teeth properly each night. The bacteria in plaque damage teeth and gums by causing tooth decay and gum disease. Plaque on the teeth can produce acid from any sugar that is taken into the mouth. This acid destroys the tooth surface leading to decalcification and eventually, tooth decay. Decalcification, the initial stage of decay, is indicated by unattractive, disheartening, and permanent white spots that are sometimes left on teeth after the brackets are removed. It is totally preventable with proper care of the teeth and braces. Plaque also releases poisons that irritate and infect the gum tissue, resulting in gum disease. New layers of plaque grow on the teeth each day. That's why plaque should be brushed from the teeth thoroughly and regularly.

Flossing during orthodontic treatment is tricky and takes a little more time, but with practice it gets easier. Flossing removes debris and food from between teeth. Since an archwire usually joins all the teeth together, floss must be threaded under the archwire first, using an aid such as a floss threader. Some types of floss come with stiffened ends that can easily be slipped under the archwire and used to guide the floss into place.

We often recommend special tools to use in brushing, such as interproximal brushes that have tiny, Christmas tree-like brushes on one end, designed to get around braces and wires. They are great for brushing between braces, with or without toothpaste.

We also recommend a water flosser (such as Waterpik), which helps flush debris from around the braces and between teeth. Sonic toothbrushes are also good at vibrating debris and bacteria off of teeth. When we see patients who use one or more of these devices routinely, we definitely see not only clean teeth but also very healthy, pink, tight gums.

Prescription-strength fluoride in gel or liquid form is also highly recommended. Fluoride helps kill germs and hardens the enamel to protect it from decalcification white spots or even cavities. The fluoride gel can be applied to the teeth with a brush or, in rinse form, can be swished around the mouth. We recommend using fluoride before bedtime after cleaning the teeth thoroughly, as nighttime is when decay-causing germs are most active.

At Depew Orthodontics, we are very attuned to the importance of good oral hygiene and take time with each appointment to examine the teeth for any signs of trouble, and we remind and reeducate patients on proper care as often as needed.

Once treatment is finished, it must be retained. That's the only way to keep a great smile.

CHAPTER NINE

Life After Braces— Wearing Your "Tooth Pajamas"

Congratulations! With your braces off, it's time to greet the world with a great smile.

One of the most important aspects of orthodontics is maintaining the teeth in the position they were in at the end of treatment. Orthodontists are perfectionists. We want teeth to be perfect and we want them to stay that way.

When patients ask how long they will have to wear retainers, my answer is, "As long as you want to have straight teeth." I like to call retainers "tooth pajamas." When it's time for bed, you brush your teeth, put on your pajamas, put on your tooth pajamas, and go to bed.

Before I talk more about

Johnny: "Doctor, how long do I have to wear retainers? Doctor: "As long as you want to have straight teeth."

retainers, let's look at some of the finishing touches we do when the braces come off.

THE FINISHING TOUCHES

When it's time to take the braces off, we first ensure the patient (and parents) are happy with the result. Usually, we know ahead of time that we're going to be removing everything, so that appointment is already scheduled.

We start by having the patients sit in the chair and bite hard on a piece of cotton to stabilize their teeth. We use special pliers to distort the bracket just a bit, which pops it off the tooth. We do one tooth at a time until all the brackets are off. Usually, the wires are still in place. But when the last bracket is removed, the whole system (brackets and wire) comes off at once.

Once the braces are off, there are other treatments that we use to complete the finishing touches. Which treatment we use depends on the patient's specific case. Other than the last one, the following procedures must all be performed by the doctor.

Cement removal is accomplished with a rotary hand piece, scaler, and polishing tools to sand off cement that remains stuck to the teeth after the brackets are removed and to polish the teeth very carefully to get back their original shine.

Laser gum contouring uses amplified, concentrated light targeted to a specific area to reshape the gum line around your teeth. Since gums often become swollen during orthodontic treatment, we can use the laser to contour the gums and create a nice, scalloped appearance so that when you smile, you show longer teeth and less gum. For more complex cases, the patient is referred to a periodontist.

Reshaping or contouring the edges of the teeth—typically, the incisors and other front teeth—can help give them a more youthful appearance. Unevenness or bumps on the edges of the teeth are more obvious once the teeth are aligned. Incisal contouring involves using a bur in a hand piece to carefully remove worn areas, chips, or developmental bumps on the edges of the teeth.

Equilibration is the selective contouring or shaping of the biting surfaces of some teeth, primarily back teeth. Equilibration is done to help the patient bite evenly on all teeth and to prevent potential interferences when the jaw is moved forward or sideways. Equilibration is not always necessary. Sometimes the doctor will let the teeth settle for a few months before doing this procedure and may require models mounted on an articulator to simulate the bite and jaw movements in order to plan the procedure in advance.

Interproximal reduction, which I mentioned in chapter eight, is the selective sanding of the interproximal surfaces, especially lower incisors, to help prevent the pressures that lead to relapse. In cases of minor post-treatment relapse, it may be done in an effort to realign the affected teeth.

Whitening is done with a product that is safe to use on adults. It is a special type of peroxide that lightens the teeth gently over time. Whitening can be done in the office with stronger chemicals or it can be done with chemical gels that the patient takes home. The home treatment uses bleaching trays that are worn with the whitening agent placed inside the trays. If you have clear plastic retainers, you can even use those in place of bleaching trays.

SHIFT HAPPENS

Teeth are not set in stone. They're sitting in living, moving, changing tissue, the bone that the teeth live in, and the gum tissue that surrounds the teeth. With that living tissue, there are natural forces in play that can cause relapse to happen.

For example, there are collagen (protein) fibers between the incisors that are stretched when teeth are moved. After braces are removed, teeth may move back toward to where they were originally, as the fibers contract back to an unstretched position. Incisors or canines that were turned before treatment may want to turn back after treatment if retention is not maintained.

Forces from the natural functioning of the lips, cheeks, and tongue also affect teeth, which are in balance between the tongue on the inside and the lips and cheeks on the outside. These muscle forces can exert significant force on the teeth, especially if this balance has been disrupted during treatment by teeth being moved too far inward or two far outward.

Typically, when the braces are removed, it's common for some teeth to remain slightly mobile for a few weeks. That is why it is important for patients to wear their retainers according to the doctor's directions. Most orthodontists have a recommended regimen for wearing retainers. Some doctors recommend full-time wear, meaning that patients are to wear the retainer day and night, except when eating or brushing their teeth. That allows the teeth to stabilize better before tapering the retention program off to nighttime wear only. Other doctors have patients go straight to nighttime wear only. The length of time the patients need to wear their retainer is determined by the doctor. In my office, we tend to have kids wear the retainers from three weeks to three months, depending on the type of retainer, full-time (day and night). Thereafter, they wear them only at night.

THE WISDOM TEETH DEBATE

There is a debate in dentistry about whether wisdom teeth cause relapse. Some say that as the wisdom teeth erupt, they push forward, causing them to push other teeth toward the front of the mouth. That can cause a relapse of teeth that have been straightened. But even after wisdom teeth have erupted, teeth naturally tend to drift toward the front of the mouth. So even if the wisdom teeth are extracted, teeth will continue to move.

The longer patients wear their retainers, the better the chance that their teeth will stay in place. Educating patients about this and encouraging them to continue wearing their retainers for as long as possible helps to minimize relapse, so we take the time to explain to patients the importance of retention in keeping their smile for a lifetime.

RETAINERS: REMOVABLE OR FIXED

The type of retainer used depends on the doctor's philosophy and experience. Proper planning for retention is the orthodontist's job and should be considered in the treatment planning stage. For example, the plan should look at avoiding expansion in cases where the pressure from normal cheek and lip activity tends to push the teeth back inward. On the other hand, treatment may avoid retracting incisors when the patient has a large, active tongue that pushes outward on the teeth. Significant movements, such as closing a big space in the teeth, or correcting the position of a tooth that was severely turned or blocked out of position, may mean looking at a more permanent type of retention once treatment is done.

Retainers fall into two main categories: 1) removable, meaning they can be put in and taken out by the patient, and 2) fixed, meaning they're attached to the teeth.

Retainers are, generally, made on a plaster model of the patient's teeth at the end of treatment. In some offices, the braces are removed in order to make an impression of one or both arches. From that, a plaster model is made and sent to a lab for the fabrication of a retainer. The patients return in a week or two to be given their retainers. If an orthodontist has an in-house lab, the retainers can be made much more quickly, often the same day or overnight, in order to avoid the risk of teeth moving during that time between the removal of the braces and retainer delivery.

An alternative method is taking the mold before the braces are fully removed and have a lab scrape the braces off the model to make the retainers so they can be delivered during the appointment when the braces are removed. That's a great way to avoid delay between the removal of the braces and retainer delivery. It can also be done very accurately using the digital process described in the next section.

Some doctors mostly use fixed retainers; others mostly use removable retainers. In my practice, we look at each case on an individual basis and determine which retainer would be best for the patient. For example, if a patient had a lot of spaces between the teeth before we moved them, I would likely recommend a removable retainer. If someone had a lot of crowding of the lower incisors before treatment, I would lean toward a fixed retainer because I know those teeth have a greater tendency to relapse.

There are pros and cons to both options.

Removable retainers are made of acrylic and wire or of clear plastic.

The conventional option for acrylic-and-wire retainers is a Hawley. This type of retainer is, basically, made of wires embedded in acrylic. The main wire is called the bow because it stretches across the front of the incisors. The acrylic is custom-molded to fit against the patient's palate on the inside of the upper jaw or the inside of the lower jaw, and wire clasps hold the retainer to the teeth. These are standard retainers that have been used for decades and they're very durable. If made properly, they can last for years and years.

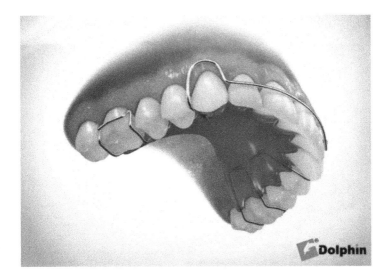

Clear plastic is another very popular type of retainer. Clear plastic retainers are less visible than other retainers because there's no wire. They're made by a procedure that heats up plastic and thermally forms it over the model of the teeth under either a high vacuum or high air pressure. In other words, they are forced down from above or sucked down from below to mold the plastic over the model of the teeth. After being allowed to cool to room temperature, they are then trimmed to create a nice, smooth edge near the gum line.

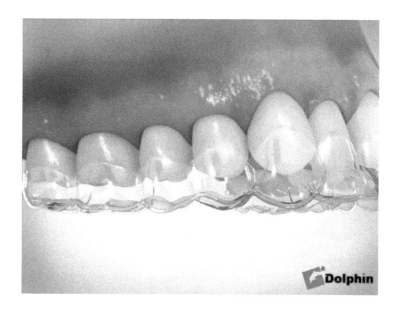

Today, in my office, our technologies such as 3-D digital impressions, an in-house lab, and 3-D printing allow us to take a scan, digitally remove the braces, and prepare a virtual model on a computer, and then we print an extremely accurate digital model. We no longer use plaster to make the tooth models for these retainers. We can make and deliver custom-made, in-house retainers on the same day that treatment is completed, saving the patient from having to schedule another appointment. This allows us to provide retainers with great efficiency and great accuracy, greatly reducing the need for molds and the use of plaster. This unique method also avoids the chance of the teeth moving if the braces are removed and the patient has to wait for the lab to receive the molds and fabricate the retainers, which can take a week or two.

Clear plastic retainers fit just to the gum line on the upper and lower teeth. Since we're able to make them in-house, we can give them to the patients the day they have their braces removed. We take the braces off, remove the bracket glue from their teeth, and, in that same session, snap in the new retainers, which fit like a glove. It's awesome to see the kinds of benefit those advances bring to our patients.

Removable retainers can be taken out for eating, cleaning, and flossing. However, the downside of removable retainers is they can be easily lost or damaged. Here are some of the more common reasons:

- **Tossed away after a meal**. You've undoubtedly heard of children or their parent dumpster-diving for lost retainers? Families go to a restaurant for a meal, the children remove the retainers to eat, wrap them in a napkin for protection, and forget about them, and then they are tossed away with the trash. It's actually a fairly frequent occurrence.

- **Lost during a swim**. We've also had patients who've lost their retainers in the ocean or pool. They get hit by a wave or are goofing off, their retainers pop out, and are gone. The clear ones are totally invisible in water.

- **The dog ate them**. Dogs love retainers too. The saliva makes the retainers a salty, tasty treat for the family pet.

- **Rigorous cleaning**. Plastic retainers are sensitive to heat. Patients who try to sterilize them by boiling them find that out quickly. They end up with a distorted glob of plastic.

- **Wear and tear**. Just as your car tires wear, so do retainers. The amount of wear depends on how much the retainers are worn and how well they're cared for. They might last two years; they might last ten years. Occasionally, retainers should be replaced if they are to remain effective as our intention is for them to be worn for many years.

- **Crunched in a pants pocket**. Retainers always come with a protective case, which is best for storing them when they're not on the teeth. But without a case handy, patients will sometimes place them in a pocket—with disastrous results.

- Grinding/chewing. People who grind their teeth tend to damage clear retainers on a regular basis. For grinders, we suggest either the standard Hawley-type retainers or a customized bite guard.

Removable retainers can develop buildups of food debris, plaque, and even tartar. Therefore, they should be cleaned at least once per day with a toothbrush, water, and liquid hand soap (toothpaste will dull the shine). There are also some commercially available products that retainers can be soaked in to keep them clean and bright. Soaking them in a mint-flavored mouthwash can also keep them smelling fresh. But beware. They might pick up the color of the mouthwash.

Fixed Retainers

Fixed retainers generally involve having a small wire bonded to the back of the front teeth, usually the six lower front teeth, and either two, four, or six upper front teeth. Since they are on the back of the teeth, they are very well hidden from view, but always working.

Just as braces do, fixed retainers require a little more care when eating. Crunchy and sticky foods and bad habits such as chewing on pencils or fingernails can break the bonds off the teeth. Although you don't have to be quite as careful as you would be with regular braces, it's still good to consider the list of foods to avoid or be careful about, mentioned in chapter eight.

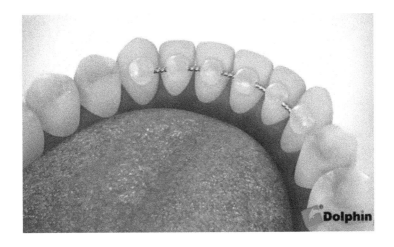

It's very important to floss regularly to keep the retainers clean, just as you would with braces, because plaque and food can become lodged under the wire and between the teeth. Without that extra attention, the plaque turns into hardened tartar, which can only be removed by a dental hygienist.

Since the wire is stretched from tooth to tooth behind the teeth, there are special brushing and flossing instructions for fixed retainers. Ideally, these steps should be done as part of a daily routine. Here are the instructions we give patients:

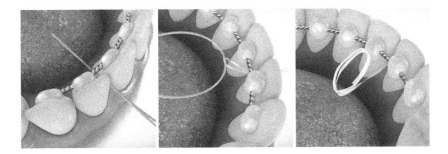

- Use a floss threader and about twelve inches of floss.

- Place the end of the floss into the loop of the threader.

- Pass the threader just above the gum line between the two lower front teeth.

- Pull it through the space between the teeth, between the gum and retainer wire.

- Floss the side of each tooth by wrapping the floss around it and moving the floss up and down.

- Remove the floss.

- Repeat for each space the retainer goes across.

Fixed retainers can break. And when they break, adverse effects can happen quite quickly. If a fixed retainer breaks, call your orthodontist immediately to get it fixed, ideally within a few days.

FIBEROTOMY

Another option that can help with retention is circumferential fiberotomy, a very minor surgical procedure that is designed to release the collagen fibers so that the elastic force is taken away, helping to minimize relapse. Sometimes, to keep the fibers from contracting, we'll do that on teeth that were severely rotated before treatment. Once released, the fibers will reorient themselves to the tooth's new position.

RETAINERS FOR LIFE

I firmly believe that patients must wear retainers for life as a way of protecting their investment. Since retainers can be expensive to replace, we have a program that helps patients stay in retainers for a lifetime. As I mentioned in chapter three, our lifetime retainer program, known as Save My Smile, allows you to get four replacement retainers per year, forever, for an upfront fee and a small copayment at the time of replacement.

I also mentioned our Guarantee My Smile program for people who, for example, lose their retainers and don't replace them, and then their teeth start moving. Through this program, we'll re-treat the patient at a reduced cost, in a very limited way, usually focusing on a few teeth rather than the entire bite.

THE BIG DAY

When the braces come off, we have a big celebration for patients. We are excited for our patients because they are free to eat what they want and smile as big as they want. We gather staff, and any family members present, around the patient and sing a celebration song for the patient: "You got your braces off today, hurrah, hurrah! You got your braces off today, hurrah, hurrah!" We usually also present a bucket full of candy or other foods that were restricted during the treatment. And the patients are presented with a celebratory certificate. Then we cheer the patients on as they leave the office. It's a hugely important day for patients.

While treatment for most of our patients involves braces, aligners, or auxiliary appliances, there's a subcategory of patients who need other types of treatment. These are patients who have issues with either TMJ or sleep disorders.

CHAPTER TEN

A Word About TMJ and Sleep Disorders

Sometimes during an exam, we find out that a patient is dealing with problems associated with TMJ disorder or sleep disorders. These are complex issues that are challenging to fit into a busy orthodontic practice since they usually need multidisciplinary care that goes beyond orthodontics. Depending on the diagnosis, we offer some orthodontic solutions. But many of these patients are referred to providers who specialize in other therapies or even surgery.

Let me share with you some of the basics of these two issues to help you see how complex they can be.

TMJ DISORDERS

TMJ refers to the temporomandibular joint, which is located just in front of the ear on both sides of your head. It is a ball-and-socket joint, much like your hip joint, that opens and closes your jaw. Inside the joint, there is a small cartilage-like disc along with ligaments, tendons, and some vascular tissue. The tissue is very sensitive, and when it becomes inflamed it causes pain, swelling, and difficulty chewing and eating.

What's interesting about the TMJ is that when the mouth opens, it opens to about twenty millimeters as the ball, called the condyle, rotates within the socket. Then the condyle translates, or slides, down a slope called the articular eminence, and the jaw opens from about twenty millimeters to about fifty millimeters. The popping sound that is a hallmark of TMJ disorders often happens as the jaw goes from rotation to translation and the little cartilage-like disc slips out of position instead of staying in place on top of the ball portion of the socket as it moves. That forward and backward, forward and backward movement is what causes the popping sound.

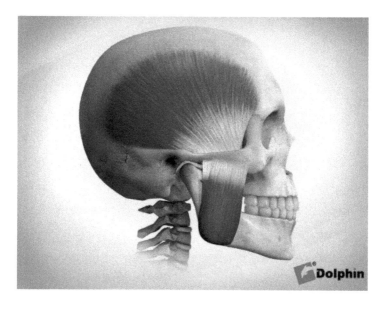

The group of TMJ problems is called TMD, or temporomandibular disorder (or dysfunction). Addressing TMD can mean addressing the joints themselves, but more often than not, it also involves the head and neck muscles involved in chewing that have become inflamed and spasmatic.

Symptoms of TMD can include pain in the joint right in front of the ear. It can be pain in any of the muscles around the mouth and in the temples, the neck, and the back of the head. It can include clicking noises in the joints, which again, come from that little cartilage-like disc moving back and forth when it's not supposed to. There's also a grating noise known as crepitus, which is when there is a misshaped disc or bone surface, or even small pieces of bone in the joint fluid. Patients also often complain of stuffiness or fullness in or around the ears. Other symptoms that are especially concerning include limited ability to open the mouth, a jaw that deviates off-center, or that is painful while opening or closing. Difficulty eating and talking, and headaches, primarily in the temple or in the back of the head, are often related to TMD.

There are multiple causes of TMD that include what are known as parafunctional habits. These habits include clenching and grinding of teeth. People who are under a lot of stress tend to clench and grind their teeth. That often happens at night, during sleep, when people aren't even aware they're doing it. Sometimes a bed partner will hear the grinding sound; sometimes even small children clench and grind. That constant clenching and grinding can distress the joints and can lead to spasm of the chewing muscles.

Trauma is another cause of TMD. A blow to the jaw can knock the disc loose, damage the joints, and cause inflammation in the joints.

A bad bite is another cause. There's a relationship between the jaw hinge, the TMJ, and the way the teeth fit. It's kind of like a three-legged stool, where the joints are two of the legs, and the teeth in contact are the third leg. A poorly functioning joint on one or both sides, and the stool falls down. Without all three legs functioning properly, things can go awry. As it relates to the bite, it could be an uneven bite or a tooth out of position that's causing the teeth to hit on one side before the other side. That can move the joint out of center and cause problems. Sometimes people will notice when they have a new filling or crown done that, after the numbness from the treatment has worn off, their bite doesn't feel right. If they clench down on it, that action can disrupt the joints. If that occurs, a quick visit to the treating dentist can usually resolve the problem.

Diagnosing TMJ and related muscle issues is complex. It involves far more than a cursory oral exam. It includes a thorough clinical evaluation of the bite, the way the jaw moves, and sounds in the joint itself. The most critical information in diagnosing TMJ issues is thoroughly discussing the symptoms, when they started, how often they happen, and how they affect the patient's day-to-day life. Besides standard orthodontic diagnostic records (photos, panoramic x-ray, cephalometric x-ray, and digital scan or impressions) we also take detailed 3-D and 2-D images of the joints, using state-of-the-art CBCT imaging, which allows us to see the joints very clearly. We also review the medical history and medications a patient may be taking. With this information, we can come up with a treatment plan for the patient or seek help from other health care providers if we feel it will be helpful.

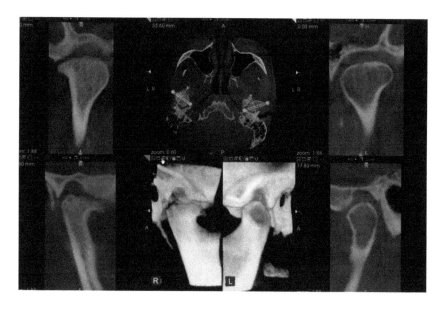

TREATMENTS FOR TMJ

As a dental professional, my job is to deal with the bite issues to ensure they're appropriate, but also create appliances to help manage the clenching and grinding. We really can't deal with the stress, which is a psychological issue outside our scope, but we can deal with how to manage the damage caused by the stress in joints and in teeth.

There are multiple treatments for TMJ that depend on the cause of the problems, the symptoms the patient is experiencing, and where the pain or dysfunction is. Just as almost anything in medicine does, the treatments depend on whom you consult. We had a joke in dental school that if you had TMJ, the treatment for it depended on which floor of the dental school you were on. So, if you were on the oral surgery floor, you needed to have surgery for your TMJ. If you were on the orthodontics floor, you needed braces. If you were on the restorative floor, you'd need to have new crowns. So, TMJ treatment depends on the symptoms but also on who helps you.

Treatments for TMJ disorders include physical therapy or massage, different types of bite guards or bite splints depending on the goal, injections of medications, arthroscopic surgery to clean the joint, or major surgery to reconstruct the joint.

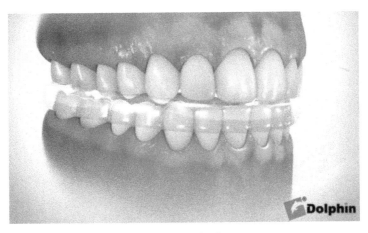

Inter-occlusal splint.

We try to treat TMJ cases very conservatively. If we catch the problem early on, it can be treated with over-the-counter medication, muscle relaxants, a soft diet, and hot and warm compresses on the joint. The next step is a bite appliance, often in conjunction with physical therapy. We often mix that with transcutaneous electrical nerve stimulation (TENS), a therapy in which electrodes are attached to the treatment area and a small jolt of energy is sent to the muscles. That jolt causes them to flex, then relax, flex, then relax. The treatment takes care of muscle spasms and helps to improve blood flow to the muscles. Using a cold laser has proven to be helpful as well.

The bite splints that are used for TMJ treatment are worn twenty-four hours a day in order to achieve relief of symptoms, and then the patient is gradually weaned off them. We will often see relief of symptoms within a few weeks or months. There are different kinds of splints with different goals. Some fit on the upper teeth, some fit on the lower teeth. When TMD is treated with a bite appliance, the bite itself can change. So, sometimes patients go through phases of treatment. The first phase is to relieve symptoms and normalize the joint, using some of the methods mentioned above, often with a splint. Once the joints and muscles are comfortable, a second phase may include braces, crowns, or jaw surgery. Other patients just stay in nighttime bite splints for the rest of their life.

Getting treatment from someone who specializes in TMJ disorders can produce great results. But it sometimes takes multiple tries, or practitioners, to get relief. There's not always one great solution.

AIRWAY AND SLEEP DISORDERS

A hot topic in health care discussions these days has to do with snoring and sleep apnea, which are sleep disorders. These tend to affect middle-age to older adults who are a little bit overweight, but they can affect people at any age or of any body type.

Airway or sleep disorders in children can lead to symptoms such as poor sleep, tiredness, exhaustion, inability to take tests properly, falling asleep at school, bedwetting, and behavioral issues. Parents often can't pinpoint that their child's problems have to do with sleep disorders, and until their child is diagnosed, parents don't know what to do.

Symptoms in adults are the same or similar and include snoring, disrupted sleep, daytime sleepiness, and brain fog. People who have sleep apnea tend to have bags under their eyes, they fall asleep easily during the daytime, and again, they tend to be overweight.

There are two kinds of sleep apnea. Central sleep apnea is more of a medical issue that can't be dealt with through dentistry. It occurs because your brain doesn't send proper signals to the muscles that control your breathing.

Obstructive sleep apnea is the more common type for which some dental treatments as well as medical remedies available. Obstructive sleep apnea is commonly caused by an obstruction of the upper airway, such as swollen nasal passages or soft tissue in the throat that collapses when the sufferers relax during sleep. With our CBCT, we can measure the airway and do some comparison evaluation on a single patient over different time periods, including before and after treatment.

Nasal passages that are blocked due to narrowness or swelling can prevent the proven benefits of nasal breathing (such as warming and filtering the air), and can also lead to obligatory mouth breathing, whether the sufferer is awake or asleep. With constant mouth breathing, there are often unhealthy changes in the oral tissues and adverse growth of the face and jaws. Typically, we'll see a narrow palate, gummy smile, and a long face. Sometimes we even see an open bite in which the front teeth cannot even touch together.

There are several orthodontic treatments available for both

children and adults.

For starters, one recommended treatment by physicians is to lose weight. That's because when sleep apnea sufferers lie on their back to sleep, the volume and weight of the tongue and surrounding tissues tend to make the tongue and surrounding tissue drop back in the throat and block the airway. Losing weight takes care of some of that volume and makes the occurrence of breathing issues less likely.

Treatments for children involve using expanders to widen the palate. Again, these improve airflow through the airway by opening the nasal passages, since the roof of the mouth is the floor of the nose. Widening the palate not only widens the nasal passages but also leaves more room for the tongue to rest forward. Myofunctional exercises to help the patient learn to breathe, swallow, and establish proper tongue and jaw posture at rest have proven helpful as well. Evaluation and treatment by an ear, nose, and throat (ENT) doctor is also often quite helpful. Oropharyngeal exercises have proven helpful for adult patients.

We can also bring the lower jaw forward to open the airway. In kids, we can bring it forward permanently through growth modification therapy, as discussed earlier in this book. In adults, we can permanently bring it forward with orthognathic surgery. However, many adults benefit from treatments that are not so drastic.

For adults, we can bring the lower jaw forward with an appliance that is worn during sleep and opens the airway by pulling the tongue and associated tissues out of the back of the throat. The appliance allows the wearer to breathe more easily throughout the night. I've created many of these for patients whose spouses say the appliances have made a world of difference. They say they sleep better because their spouse is sleeping better.

The nighttime appliance for adults is an excellent alternative to the continuous positive airway pressure (CPAP) machine that is often prescribed for sleep apnea patients. Most patients really struggle to wear the CPAP night after night. But the oral appliance is easier to wear and it helps them breathe better and get more air into their lungs. The appliance is really a Band-aid and when patients remove it in the morning after a night of sleep, their bite often feels a bit different. Simply clenching the bite together will begin to return the bite to its normal function. But long-term wear may lead to a more permanent change in the bite, requiring further treatment.

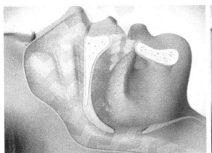
Open airway

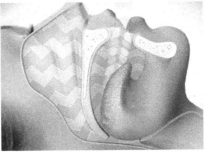
Constricted airway

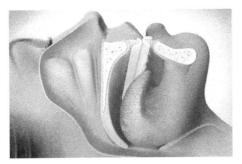
Airway with appliance

There are also surgical options for obstructive sleep apnea that are performed by ENTs and oral surgeons. These are last-resort options that we only turn to if conservative treatments don't work. An ENT can open the nasal airway, or an oral surgeon can move the lower jaw forward, and the base of the tongue along with it, to open the airway.

Sleep apnea patients are often already diagnosed before they come to us for treatment. As we do with all our patients, we evaluate them and then offer customized solutions, which again, in very complex cases, may mean referring them to another provider.

Conclusion

At Depew Orthodontics, our goal is to change lives. We have seen personalities blossom, career paths become enriched, and relationships flourish after helping our patients transform their teeth into incredible smiles.

I hope that with this book I have helped clear up some of the confusion about the orthodontic treatments and technologies available today. With so many providers to choose from, I hope that you now have some insight into what to look for to best serve yourself and your family.

It's important to find someone who will give you the level of care you deserve. Remember that orthodontists undergo extra, specialized training beyond dental school to learn how to move teeth. Then we spend our working days using that training and our skills to treat patients, choosing the best options to give them what they want and need.

One of my favorite orthodontic experiences is seeing all the amazing technology that allows us to more accurately diagnose patients and create a customized digital treatment plan. The technologies make for a far better experience for the patient than ever before.

But it's not just about the tools; it's primarily the hands guiding those tools that make the difference. As an orthodontic specialist with nearly three decades of experience, I know how orthodontic treatment can change your life.

And that's what it's all about. My primary goal is to respect the individual needs and wants of patients while providing the highest quality orthodontic care in a pleasing and friendly environment. Together, my team and I strive every day to create for our patient family the winning smiles that will last them a lifetime.

About the Author

Dr. Doug Depew has maintained a thriving orthodontic practice in Cobb County, Georgia, since 1990. He graduated magna cum laude from the University of Georgia and was ranked at the top of his dental school class in all of the four years he studied at the Medical College of Georgia. He earned his certificate in orthodontics and master's degree from Baylor College of Dentistry at Baylor University. Today, he is active in the American Association of Orthodontists, the Southern Association of Orthodontists, the Georgia Association of Orthodontists, the American Lingual Orthodontic Association, the Spear Dental Study Club, and the Elite Lingual Orthodontic Society.

Dr. Depew is also the founder and academic director of Trapezio, an innovative, online program endorsed by the American Association of Orthodontists (AAO) and recognized internationally as the standard for training and certification of orthodontic staff members. As the program creator, Dr. Depew is frequently invited to speak at professional meetings around the country and overseas.

As leader of the Depew Orthodontics team, Dr. Depew oversees a team of highly trained dental and orthodontic professionals who take great pride in their work and are dedicated to making patients feel comfortable and excited about their orthodontic experience. Depew Orthodontics is the only practice in its area that has been granted the Academy of Orthodontic Assisting's Gold Certification and the prestigious designation of 3M Center of Excellence.

Our Services

Welcome to Depew Orthodontics!

At Depew Orthodontics, our goal is to change lives—period. We have seen personalities blossom, career paths become enriched, and relationships flourish after helping our patients transform their teeth into incredible smiles. We truly feel that our patients are our family and do all we can to help them feel welcome and excited to be here with us. We pride ourselves on providing patients and family members with a warm and comfortable environment. We believe our patients are special, and we prove it every time they visit our office.

We are known for giving the most thorough and informative initial orthodontic consultations, and that initial appointment is offered at no charge for those looking to start wearing braces or aligners.

During that visit, we evaluate your smile and bite, assess and discuss your concerns, and review a customized orthodontic treatment plan with you, along with any options or alternatives you may have.

We specialize in providing quality orthodontic treatment for children, teens, and adults, and have the training, technology, and techniques to give you the most advanced care. We're a leading provider of Clarity ceramic braces, Incognito braces, SmartClip appliances, and

Invisalign clear aligners. And we have the most flexible financing plans available to make treatment affordable for anyone.

At our office, you are more than just a patient. You are family!

Our complimentary Brace Bus service, picking up children from school for their appointments, is an example of our over-the-top customer service.

Our entire staff is trained through Trapezio, an online program endorsed by the American Association of Orthodontists and recognized internationally as the standard for orthodontic staff training and certification.

At our office, you are more than just a patient. You are family!

FOR MORE INFORMATION

Visit us at www.depewsmiles.com.

For for information bout Trapezio,
visit www.trapezio.com.

Kennesaw

2748 Watts Drive, Kennesaw, Georgia 30144
Phone: 770-422-3939 office@depewsmiles.com

Cedarcrest

2161 Cedarcrest Road, Acworth, Georgia 30101
Phone: 770-422-3939 office@depewsmiles.com

Atlanta

1820 The Exchange S.E., Atlanta, Georgia 30339
Phone: 770-952-2677 office@depewsmiles.com